Praise for
Crash: A Memoir of Overmedication and Recovery

"Ann Bracken's evocative memoir powerfully tells of how psychiatry's diagnoses and treatments can lead to loss, illness, and despair, and how escaping from that paradigm of care can be a starting point for a full and robust recovery."
Robert Whitaker, author of *Anatomy of an Epidemic*

"Ann Bracken artfully braids her path out of chronic pain and major depression, while questioning the system designed to help her, and reaching back into her mother's history to find a way to help her as well. Bracken gives us permission to ask questions about our current mental health treatment; read and educate ourselves on the risks, benefits, and alternatives to psychiatry's status quo; and above all, not to quit until we find our own path to a healed life."
Angela Peacock, MSW, mental health advocate and featured in award-winning documentary, *Medicating Normal*

"A fascinating memoir of two generations of medical and psychiatric mismanagement and suffering, and how one brave woman figured out what was happening and successfully took control of her health and well-being... and prevented a third generation from following the same path."
Stuart Shipko, MD, author of *Surviving Panic Disorder* and *Xanax Withdrawal*.

"Crash is a beautifully written memoir of intergenerational struggle... Informed by deeply personal experiences and careful research, Bracken clearly illustrates just how much "help" can sometimes hurt, particularly when it is filtered through the arrogance endemic to our treatment systems."
**Sera Davidow, Director at The Wildflower Alliance:
A Grassroots Peer Support, Advocacy, and Training Organization**

"In Crash: A Memoir of Overmedication and Recovery, Ann Bracken tells a gripping but all too common story of the damage that can be done by psychiatric drugs and electroconvulsive therapy. Both mother and daughter are repeatedly let down by a mental health system that is so clearly reliant on simplistic bio-medical approaches to the complex problems of life and which is unable to acknowledge the dark side of those treatments, especially for women."
Dr. John Read, Professor of Clinical Psychology, University of East London

Crash

A Memoir of Overmedication and Recovery

Ann Bracken
Charing Cross Press
Simpsonville

Also by Ann Bracken

The Altar of Innocence

No Barking in the Hallways: Poems from the Classroom

Once You're Inside: Poems Exploring Incarceration

Crash: A Memoir of Overmedication and Recovery is a view of some events in the author's life told as truthfully as recollection permits. It reflects the author's present remembrances of experiences over time, with some support from medical records, a personal journal, and records from the author's father. With the exception of the author's first name, all names, place names, and most characteristics have been changed to respect privacy, some events have been compressed, and some dialogue has been recreated.

This book is not intended as a substitute for the medical advice of physicians. The reader should consult a physician in matters relating to his/her health and particularly if the reader is considering discontinuing psychiatric drugs or pain medication. A list of organizations to assist with the withdrawal process is included in the Appendix.

Copyright © 2023 by Ann Bracken

Charing Cross Press

Charing Cross Press
All rights reserved. No part of this book may be reproduced or transmitted in any other form or by any means, electronic or mechanical, including photocopying, recording, or by any other information storage or retrieval system.

Library of Congress Control Number: 2022905148
ISBN 978-0-578-39433-6 Paperback

Cover Design: Christine Rains
Book Design: David Saunier
Logo Design: Christella Potts

Dedication

To my parents for their unfailing courage and love, to my children who always offer encouragement and support for my writing, and to my energy healer who helped me find my way back to health.

Acknowledgements

I wish to personally thank the following people for their contributions to my inspiration and knowledge and other help in creating this book:

Desiree Magney and Barbara Morrison, my first memoir instructors, Lisa Biggar for her skillful editing and encouragement, Rachel Hicks for her superb copyediting, Christine Rains and David Saunier for cover design and book layout, Patricia VanAmburg and Michele Mason for their work as beta readers, Grace Cavalieri for believing in my story, and my cousin, John Wetzler, for gifting me with the title.

Table of Contents

Introduction	1
Prologue	5
Chapter 1: Where's Mom?	7
Chapter 2: Reflections	15
Chapter 3: Just Like Your Mother	19
Chapter 4: More is Better, But No One Mentioned the Side Effects	33
Chapter 5: He'll Never Do to Me What He Did to My Mother	41
Chapter 6: Looking for the Why	47
Chapter 7: The Long Way Around	49
Chapter 8: I Never Thought I'd Do This	63
Chapter 9: If It's Not Working, Do More of It	71
Chapter 10: Getting with the Program	77
Chapter 11: ECT—the Backstory	85
Chapter 12: Down the Rabbit Hole Looking for Relief	89
Chapter 13: The Treatment-Resistant Patient	97
Chapter 14: A Therapeutic Environment	101
Chapter 15: Slow-walking to the Inevitable	111
Chapter 16: From Pollyanna to Polypharmacy	123
Chapter 17: Trust Your Inner Voice	133
Chapter 18: Why Didn't My Doctors Warn Me?	139
Chapter 19: Paradigm Shift	143
Chapter 20: What Could a Patient Possibly Understand About Clinical Trials?	153
Chapter 21: You Have a Damaged Brain	157
Chapter 22: The Book of Revelation	167
Chapter 23: Hidden in Plain Sight	175
Chapter 24: Answers Regarding Recovery—It's Complicated	181
Chapter 25: The Answers in the Attic	191
Appendix	203
Notes	211
References	221

Introduction

Have you ever survived a tragedy that turned out to be your greatest gift? Have you ever defied authority figures because you had a strong hunch that you were right? Have you ever done everything a doctor told you, only to find yourself sicker than before you began treatment?

If you can answer yes to even one of these questions, then you've opened the right book.

Maybe you're one of the millions of Americans suffering from relentless chronic pain, despite taking large amounts of powerful drugs. Every day that you decide to go on with your life is an act of courage. Sometimes you feel like your spouse or your doctors don't listen to what you're saying. Perhaps you're afraid they'll give up on you, and you'll sink into a morass of pain for the rest of your life.

Maybe you're part of the 30 to 50 percent of Americans who take a variety of psychiatric meds, yet none of the drugs, in any combination, have worked for you. Now when you visit your doctor, they tell you that you're "treatment resistant," as if you don't want to get well. Perhaps they've recommended electroconvulsive therapy (ECT), and you're almost desperate enough to agree.

Maybe you grew up in a home where one of your parents

suffered with depression, so you figure that your condition is hereditary. Have doctors told you that you have a chemical imbalance in your brain, or that once you find the right drug, you'll come back into the light?

Have you begun to question all of these ideas? Maybe you have a small voice inside promising, *Hold on to hope. The right door is nearby.*

I know that something better is possible for you because in the early 1990s, I answered *yes* to all of those questions. I was a mom in my forties with two adolescent kids and my own business when a daily, unrelenting migraine gripped me and refused to let go for seven years. And during four of those years, I also battled profound, suicidal depression.

I willingly tried every medicine and treatment my doctors recommended, but grew more despondent with every drug that failed to beat back the blackest feelings I could imagine. Even worse, when I insisted that my migraine was just one more in a series of mysterious pains that turned out to be a form of depression, the doctors shut me out. Hoping for relief from at least one of the agonizing conditions I was living with, I eagerly filled the prescription when a new headache doctor told me that the drug called OxyContin was safe and non-addictive—and would surely finish off my headache.

I wrote this book because from 1993 to 2000, I struggled to find my way out of depression and chronic pain. I stood up to my husband when he repeatedly told me, "You're just like your mother—you'll never get well." And I was determined to prove him wrong. As the poet Mary Oliver put it, I was "…determined to save / the only life [I] could save"

I also wrote this book to explore my mother's experience with depression and chronic pain, and to put forward a plausible story of why she never recovered. Up until I found thirty years' worth of my father's detailed records of her care, my hypothesis was that Mom self-medicated with alcohol along with taking many psychiatric drugs—a very dangerous and destructive combination.

But Dad's records laid out a more detailed and nuanced reason for my mother's suffering. And as I researched her care and compared it to mine, I found that despite its claims to the contrary, psychiatry had progressed very little from 1959 to 2000 in providing successful, humane treatments for people like Mom and me.

I hope this introduction has piqued your interest. Come along with me on my journey to healing and share in the truth of my story. And maybe you'll even discover a successful resolution for your challenges.

Prologue

"Lady, are you all right?" I woke up suddenly. A man in a dark leather jacket pounded on my driver's side window.

A pungent smell filled the car. I felt the airbag pushing me up against my seat, wedging me in place. *Must wake up.* The man pounded on the window again. I rolled it down and looked at him through heavy-lidded eyes.

"I'm so drugged."

"Lady, don't ever say that again."

The cold air rushing into the car jolted me awake. What had happened? I saw a black van stopped inches away from the front of my car. Traffic crawled and then crept past us. I was pinned behind the airbag, but, somehow, I managed to free myself and get out of the car. We stood in the middle of Route 40, the main thoroughfare through Baltimore, surveying the damage. The man's van didn't have a scratch on it, but the front of my little Toyota was pretty banged up.

Before I could ask him any questions, he ordered me back into my car. "Park in one of those empty spaces," he directed, motioning to the lot next to our crash site. He hopped into his van and led me to a parking spot.

I think the man in the dark jacket asked me if I was all right, but I was dazed, or more likely, in a stupor. I expected him to be angry, but, instead, he patiently waited in the cold with me. I can't remember if I had a cell phone, but I must have. Did I give it to the man and ask him to call my father? Maybe.

In a few minutes my dad arrived, and I think he talked to the man in the dark jacket. Dad hugged me and wanted to know if I was OK. *At least he wasn't angry with me.*

What just happened? No one had been hurt, but my car was banged up. *Randy's going to kill me*, echoed through my thoughts, when I imagined the inevitable confession to my husband. My neck began to hurt, but I don't think I cried.

"I have to give that man my insurance information," I told Dad, and fumbled in the glove compartment, looking for the documents. But when I found them and got out of the car, the man in the dark jacket was gone. He never asked for my name or phone number. To this day, I swear he was an angel.

"Come on home, Ann. We'll talk there and get you warmed up," Dad said.

Still dazed, I wondered *Am I in shock?* I remember going to my parents' house and having tea with them. Their calm demeanors and kind words masked any worry they may have felt.

As I sat in the yellow kitchen, both hands cupped around the steaming tea mug, I began to piece together the events of that afternoon. My mind raced as my parents' voices faded into the background. I knew that people walked in between cars all the time on Route 40, especially when traffic was stopped. What if a pedestrian had been between the van and my car? At the very least, I could have hurt someone badly. Was I going fast or had I slowed down? There must have been some momentum for the airbag to explode like that. Maybe I fell asleep before I put on the brakes? *Oh, God, I could have killed someone.* And like every other drunk or drug addict, I would walk away without an injury. And someone else would pay for my carelessness.

Chapter 1: Where's Mom?

I'd just turned seven in June of 1959 and had devoured all of the books on my bookshelf, so Dad and I made weekly library treks to keep me stocked, and I'd curl up with them for hours on the black and white striped couch in the basement club room. I snuggled under a heavy, musty-smelling quilt that was hand-stitched out of velvets, silks, and cottons, each piece joined to the next with rainbow-colored embroidery stitches.

"It's called a crazy quilt, Ann," Mom said, as I ran my fingers over the odd-shaped scraps of silk, corduroy, and velvet. "My grandmother made it many years ago, when I was a little girl like you." She put her arm around me and squeezed me close to her. "One day I'll teach you how to make these pretty embroidery stitches," she promised.

I remember brushing the velvet against my cheek as I read and imagining the great-grandmother I never knew. Sitting there alone in the basement with my books, I thought that the best thing that had happened to my family was the birth of my baby sister Kelly in March. But right after my birthday in June, the worst thing happened—my mother disappeared.

Pieces of life occur in families when kids go off to school or when they spend all day playing outside, or when they go to bed and have to keep the door closed. Mom must have been struggling much more than my younger siblings—Moira and Rory—and I had any clue about. Our older brother, Henry, was nineteen and had left the year before for the seminary. He came home that May after his classes were over. I mostly remember him up in his room listening to the soundtrack from *The King and I* or *South Pacific* and going out with his friends in the evening. Henry and Mom were very close because he'd been the only child for twelve years before I was born.

They often walked together and sometimes went down to the basement where it was cool so they could talk. Henry remembers one day Mom was so upset that she banged her head against the wall and said, "I can't take it anymore."

I hurt inside every time I close my eyes and remember what my mother looked like—how beautiful she was, with her curly brown hair and her green eyes sparkling when she smiled. I remember Mom teaching me how to ride a two-wheeled bike on the sidewalk in front of our house.

With her hand on the bike to steady and guide me, Mom said, "It's OK to wiggle the handlebars a little till you get the hang of it." At some point, she took her hands away and I zigged and zagged down the street, until I finally fell off and scraped my knee. Mom was right there when I needed her, reassuring me. "Ann, look how far you made it. We'll go clean up your knee and try again tomorrow."

When I close my eyes and snuggle under the crazy quilt, I can still hear her calming voice. I see her wearing one of her favorite dresses when Dad took her out to dinner. I remember watching her as she dabbed perfume behind her ears and on the inside of her wrists. But somehow, I never saw her pain.

I noticed amber-colored pill bottles from Dr. S. lining one of the counters in the kitchen, but I had no idea what they were and how they were supposed to help Mom. I remember only the lazy days under the crazy quilt, holding my baby sister, and celebrating my seventh birthday with Mom's chocolate cake.

"Your mother is going away for a while," Dad told us one day. But he didn't say why. What had happened that she needed to leave? She seemed to be fine, reading to us at bedtime and making all of our meals. When I think back on those early months after Kelly's birth, I see my mother nursing the baby in a darkened room while rocking rhythmically in a creaky wooden chair. Sitting on the spare bed across from her, I lifted my blouse and put a doll to my chest, pretending to nurse. Sometimes Mom let me hold Kelly, but only if I cradled her in a pillow on my lap. "Be still, Ann, and don't let her head slip," Mom cautioned. Pictures that I have from that time show smiling parents and excited siblings, eager to help care for the baby.

And then Grandma, Mom's mother, moved in. Before Dad left for work one morning, Grandma walked into the house carrying two suitcases and installed herself in Kelly's room on the first floor. She hung her dresses in the closet and arranged her Merle Norman cosmetics and satin jewelry case on the dressing table. Moira, Rory, and I pressed Dad for an explanation: "Your grandmother's staying for a while to help with Kelly," he said before heading out the door. My mind buzzed with a million questions, but Dad's furrowed brows and tight jaw served as a red flag indicating he wouldn't tolerate any discussion.

While I have no recollection of what led up to Mom leaving, I can see myself trailing Grandma around the house as she tidied things or folded laundry. Long after my younger siblings found something to do outside, I pestered her with questions.

"Where's Mom? Why did she go away? When's she coming home, Grandma?"

"Curiosity killed the cat," Grandma said. I thought that was a strange answer because the Catholic sisters in school prized curiosity, especially when they wanted us to learn something new.

After weeks of dogging Grandma about Mom's whereabouts, I finally guessed where she could be. I made an X with my body—arms planted on hips and legs spread wide—and stood in front of her as she hurried toward the kitchen.

"I know where Mom is. She's at Uncle Chet's farm, isn't she?" Our uncle had a small farm in a neighboring county, and we'd visit every summer, enjoying hours of jumping into piles of hay and chasing chickens. Grandma sighed as I blocked her, signaling that I'd won a small victory.

"Yes, she's there, but you can't visit her."

"Can we call her?"

"No," Grandma said. "She needs rest."

Afraid I'd hear that line about curiosity killing the cat again, I decided not to ask why Mom needed to relax. "Can we write to her?" Grandma nodded, brushed her hands on her apron, and headed into the kitchen to make dinner.

I remember being schooled in the art of letter-writing, sitting at the dining room table with Mom as she penned notes to her sister and brothers who lived far away. She gathered her blue stationary, stamps, and envelopes and then told me, "Use your neatest handwriting and try to write in a straight line." I was just learning to write in cursive, and my letters were much bigger than Mom's, but I wrote a few sentences—all sloping upwards—to my cousin Sally. "That's a good start, Ann," Mom said. "Keep practicing."

That lesson with Mom was fresh in my mind later that evening as I corralled Moira and Rory to write a letter to Mom. We drew pictures of flowers and trees—things Mom loved—and filled a couple of notebook pages with our best handwriting. *We love you, Mom. We miss you. Please write back.* Dad promised to deliver our pleadings the next time he visited. Still, no one gave us any information about Mom.

Every family chooses a room where people go for private conversations, and in our house, the kitchen was the spot for sharing secrets. I remember Dad coming home from his work as a supervisor in a chemical lab at what he euphemistically called "the power company"—The Metro Power and Light Company—one day and motioning for Grandma to join him in the kitchen while the three of us watched TV. The bolting of the lock on the kitchen door cued us that secrets were about to happen. Moira, Rory, and I tiptoed into the dining room and pressed our ears to the door. The loud hum of the window air conditioner distorted the grown-ups' conversation. I remember hearing a story of what sounded like someone being nervous and someone breaking down. I remember hearing Dad say that he hoped she'd be all right. I remember the three of us praying for our mother to come home.

I can't recall Dad telling us that Mom was in a hospital, but I'm sure we wore him down enough that he confessed. Maybe that was all the explanation we needed to convince us that she needed to rest—you went to a hospital if you were sick and usually stayed in bed. I don't remember letters from Mom, but Dad brought us news when he visited her every Sunday.

Later in the summer, Dad arranged a home-visit for Mom after they had gone out to dinner. "You kids be good and don't upset your mother," he told us before he left. The afternoon passed as if we were living in a slow-motion universe while we kept a vigil on the front porch steps of our cozy brick house. When the blue Plymouth finally made its way to our driveway, we rushed Mom, covering her with hugs and kisses. I remember thinking that she was as beautiful as a queen in her dress and pearls. And like a queen, she seemed untouchable and fragile. Mindful of Dad's warning, we knew we had to behave. We thought, as Dad and Grandma had told us, if we worked to be the best kids ever, Mom would come home for good. Seeing her made me ache for her presence even more. Dad took a picture of all of us kids crowded around Mom as she sat on one of the easy chairs. She had a big smile on her face and she looked happy, so I wasn't sure why she went back to the hospital.

I was the oldest at home, so Grandma and Dad expected me to complete my schoolwork by myself, bring Rory back if he ran away at mealtimes, and help out with basic chores like setting the table and folding diapers. They heaped praise on me for being such a "big girl," but I was only seven and desperately worried about my mother. Still, no one told me anything about how she was doing or when she might come home. Secrets and whispers hung over our house as thick and heavy as Baltimore's humidity.

For a time, I was plagued with stomachaches every morning when I went to school. Sitting at my desk, wearing my blue uniform jumper and white blouse, I would clutch my stomach and wish the pain away. Grandma and Dad had no sympathy for tummy aches, and mine was no exception. But I must have complained for several weeks, so Dad gave in and took me to the pediatrician. I climbed up onto the examining table and lifted my shirt while the doctor listened to my heart and my lungs, looked in my mouth, checked my ears, felt my glands, and pressed on my stomach. He asked Dad a few questions, shone a light in my eyes, and then pronounced his diagnosis: "She needs to eat more breakfast."

After months of being in the hospital and a number of what must have been successful home-visits, Mom came home to our comfortable brick house for good in late November—well after Moira and I had started in our new grades, so we had our routines in place for school and homework. Grandma went home, but she came to help Mom with the chores and the baby a few days a week. We sensed Mom's fragility by observing how the adults cushioned everything around her—stopping by with a pot of soup or taking all of us to play at their houses for the day. Grandma's presence was enough to signal that Mom wasn't quite up to her role. And if we happened to "slip" and squabble over things, Dad issued a warning that froze all of us into submission: "You kids better behave, or you'll send your mother back to the hospital."

Obedience was very important in my family, so after Mom came home, we dutifully followed Dad's new routines. He got us up for school, made breakfast for everyone, and supervised us making our lunches. "Your mother didn't sleep well last night," he often said when Mom didn't make our breakfast or even kiss us goodbye as we left for school. Mom took a nap every day, but she managed to greet us when we came home. I remember late afternoons in the kitchen where we all sat around the red Formica table, snacking on cookies while we sipped hot tea with milk. Mom made dinner every night and read us a story before tucking us in.

All the adults in my life drank cocktails every night before dinner, but Mom was the only person I knew who drank wine. I remember Mom's wine as being very important to her, but I didn't know why. One day when I was in the basement playing, I walked around the corner and spied Dad pouring water into one of Mom's gallon-sized jugs of white wine. His hands shook when he caught sight of me, and he stopped what he was doing. I bit my lip and squished my eyebrows together as I stood watching him. "Don't ever tell your mother what you saw," he ordered. I nodded, but couldn't wait to run outside and get away. Why was he doing that? And why would he ask me to keep a secret from Mom? I felt as if I were swinging higher and higher, caught between my parents, afraid to jump.

Chapter 2: Reflections

Looking back on those fateful months in 1959, I know Dad must have seen how much Mom struggled adjusting to life with a new baby, probably compounded by her age—forty-five—and the closeness of the other three children—seven, five, and four. And while she was able to mask her distress in front of us kids, Mom must have been in desperate straits for Dad to call a psychiatrist, because the whole notion of mental illness was shrouded in layers of secrecy and shame. And if you uttered the word at all, you whispered it: *depression*.

Many years after both Mom and Dad had passed away, I discovered a trove of documents that provided missing pieces of the puzzle regarding my mother's illness and treatment. As I opened the thick file, I found a 1983 letter providing a detailed listing of drugs and treatments that Dad had shared with Dr. L., her newest doctor. In the second paragraph, Dad listed all the pills that Mom's first psychiatrist, Dr. S., prescribed for her in that six-week period in 1959 when she first became so ill: Ritalin (stimulant)[1], Nardil and Tofranil (antidepressants)[2], Trilafon (an antipsychotic)[3], Nembutal (barbiturate)[4], and Dexamyl (combination amphetamine and barbiturate)[5]. Apparently, the drugs didn't help and Dad stated in the letter, "By the end of May '59 she was so bad, that even to my nonprofessional eye, I didn't see how she could avoid hospitalization." Mom hung on for another three weeks, and was finally admitted only after Dad took it upon himself to visit the hospital and inquire about care, treatments, and rates. All of this turmoil rumbled outside of my conscious awareness.

My stomach twisted into a tight knot as I read the list of drugs my mother had consumed in such a brief period of time. Over the next few days, I dug into research and uncovered information about the many effects of the pills. Trilafon and Tofranil could both cause insomnia, Tofranil could also cause anxiety, and Ritalin could cause aggression, nervousness, and irritability. Nembutal and Nardil could result in shakiness, dizziness, and confusion. No wonder Mom had banged her head on the wall and told Henry she couldn't take it anymore.

When I think back to the stomachache incident with my pediatrician, I wonder if he knew that Mom was in a hospital. And what did he know about *my* life, as a child—a little girl who felt as if she'd lost her mother? But in the late fifties, I don't think there was much awareness of how feelings could affect one's health, and certainly not in relation to children. I believe that at some level, I'd internalized the family rule not to show emotions, especially anxiety and fear. I understood that it was OK to feel sick to my stomach, but it was not OK to cry a lot and act worried about my mother. At seven years of age, I had my first experience of my feelings talking to my body—but I didn't understand the language.

Over the next few months of that summer, I pieced together the story of Mom's disappearance. I learned that she'd been a patient in a small, Catholic, psychiatric hospital in Baltimore, not a visitor on a farm, and that her mysterious illness was called depression. The grown-ups in my life rarely said the "d" word aloud and instead used euphemisms like, "Helen's having a rough spell," or "Helen needs more rest...with the new baby and all." We internalized the unspoken rules about describing what was wrong with Mom and told our friends that sometimes she was sick.

After Mom came home, all of us kids were subjected to some bruising humor about who was responsible for her illness. One particularly dark joke loops through my memory because it happened so frequently. Dad would start out by saying, "You know your mother was fine until Ann was born—that's the first time she got sick." Everyone would laugh, because, of course, Dad was just kidding. Sometimes my cheeks flamed as my chin trembled, and I'd hang my head. Then Dad would pull back a little and say, "You know I'm kidding. Your mother and I were thrilled to have you when we saw you on that little pink blanket in the hospital." But that tale coupled with Dad's admonitions that "You kids better behave or you'll send your mother back to the hospital" instilled in us a sense of collective responsibility for Mom's suffering. After everyone got a good laugh about me, one of us, usually Rory, would say, "But Kelly really did her in. Mom was so sick after Kelly was born that she landed in a hospital." As Kelly got older, she played along, earning the tag of "a good sport" probably because she saw what happened to me when I "couldn't take a joke." I cringe at how much that story must have hurt her, and I've apologized for ever participating in that cruel family ritual.

Chapter 3: Just Like Your Mother

Life seems simple when you're a child—the sun sets, and you go to bed. The sun rises, and you get up. Likewise, if you get sick, you also get well. And all of us believed that Mom would get well, especially if we worked hard to behave and said lots of prayers. Because we'd internalized the idea that we were at least partly responsible for her illness, we knew that we'd better do what we could to be part of the cure.

But Mom's illness didn't go away. Instead, her life took on a rhythm like a roller coaster—long pulls up the hill from sadness and lethargy followed by short bursts of energy, filled with visiting friends and decorating projects around the house. And like the roller coaster in the amusement park, the downhill times were fraught with fear and a sense of impending disaster. Sometimes, Mom stayed at the bottom of the hill for a very long time, no matter how many prayers we said or how many nice things we did to cheer her up.

Bringing a new friend home involved creative thinking on my part. I knew I'd have to justify why the curtains were drawn in the living room, but worst of all, I'd have to explain why the telephone sat perched on a pillow in the dining room. I became practiced at assuming a matter-of-fact approach: "My mom takes a nap every day, so she closes the curtains to keep the house dark and puts the phone on a pillow so the ringer won't wake her up." No one ever questioned me even though I'm sure nothing like that went on in their houses, at least not the ones I visited. Because I was never certain when Mom would get up from her nap, I'd lead my friend into the kitchen so we could have a snack. I could feel all of my muscles relax as soon as Mom appeared, greeting my new friend and serving us tea and cookies.

Besides being able to take a joke and keep our feelings under control, Dad made it very clear that we weren't supposed to talk about Mom's illness. And we were never to use the word *depression*. I could add one more rule to that list—to never tell Mom that I saw Dad mixing water into her wine. What made all of those rules confusing, especially the one about keeping Mom's illness a secret and avoiding the word *depression*, was that my relatives and my parents' close friends clearly knew what was going on, because I often heard them whispering in the kitchen with Dad.

When I was about ten years old, he announced that he'd bought a pool membership—like so many of my classmates in the neighborhood—for the family, and we were all going to be able to swim every day. The unspoken part of that statement was what I heard him share on the phone with Henry and Grandma: "Helen needs a break from the kids during the summer; Ann can take them to the pool."

Getting to the pool was another story. While many of the families in the neighborhood had two cars or a father who carpooled a few days a week so his wife could have a car, Dad drove to work every day. He said, "You kids walk to school all year. You can walk to the pool, and I'll pick you up on my way home from work." And walk we did—at least two miles along a busy street and then through tree-shaded neighborhoods, up and down hills until we reached the pool. Once we arrived, we showed our membership card, changed into our swimsuits, and dove into the cool, blue water.

We were too young to sit on the wooden loungers arranged just outside the fenced pool, so we spread out our towels on the grass and ate our snacks during the fifteen minutes every hour devoted to adult swim. A tableau pops into my mind when I think about those steamy summer afternoons. Mom's friends, "the swimming pool ladies" as I christened them, regularly commandeered a group of wooden loungers that we passed by on our way to and from the water. Many of their kids were our friends, so we knew the moms quite well. They smiled at us and chatted politely, but as soon as they thought we were out of earshot, I heard things like "Those poor children—here all alone" and "I hear Helen's having a bad spell again…it's such a shame what happened to her." As if I didn't miss my mother enough or feel glaringly peculiar being the only child at the pool without a parent, I also had to endure their pitying looks and whispered gossip on a regular basis. Diving into the deep water as soon as the adult swim ended, I ached for my mother to meet me at the other end.

On the weekends, the whole family went to the pool. Eager to impress our parents, we showed them all of the dives, strokes, and tricks we'd perfected during the week. Mom smiled and clapped for us, but didn't join us in the water. Instead, we heeded Dad's warnings not to bother her so she could enjoy the peace and quiet of the adult swim. "The swimming pool ladies" welcomed Mom, offering her one of the lounge chairs or getting her a snack from the concession stand. Wherever Mom went, I noticed that her friends hovered protectively. It looked to me that they'd somehow internalized the same message that we kids knew: Don't do anything to trouble Helen so as not to set her back.

Sometimes when Dad and I were alone in the kitchen, he'd close the door and almost whisper, "I'm sorry that you kids don't know who your mother used to be." I'd wait, leaning toward him so he'd share his secrets. "Did you know that your mother used to play tennis all the time?" I couldn't imagine her having enough energy to move around a tennis court. "She always dressed stylishly, no matter where she went." Stylish? Mom's clothes were the same week after week then, to the point where I called the green- and gold-striped dress she wore every Sunday her "church dress." She had a trim figure, even after bearing five children, but she rarely wore anything other than what were called "housedresses" at the time.

Henry also told me stories about Mom from before the time I was born—before she got sick. "Mom used to be the president of her alumnae association. She always had great dinner parties and made artistic centerpieces." All I could think was that Mom must have been amazing—beautiful, competent, athletic—and we all prayed for her recovery. I pinned my hopes on the magic of doctors and pills to restore Mom to the woman everyone longed to see.

Dad did whatever he could to help Mom recover and get back to her old self. He shopped for the groceries, working from Mom's detailed lists, and bought clothes for us from Montgomery Ward when he stopped in the "Bargain Basement" on his way home from work. He attended the parent-teacher conferences and signed us up for activities in the summer so Mom could have some semblance of a routine. He took Mom out to dinner ever few weeks, and even acquiesced when she tucked a mini of gin into her purse to strengthen her martini. I guess he was more focused on controlling her daily drinking, limiting her to a cocktail before dinner and measuring out a partial decanter of wine every night to help her sleep.

Dad devoted himself to record-keeping, and I have vivid memories of him sitting at his desk at night, creating spread-sheets with his slide-rule and a red pen. "I'm keeping track of my stocks so you kids can have money to go to college," he'd tell us. Dad recorded the pertinent information regarding the purchase price, the current value, and the trend, then acted like a broker, deciding when to buy or sell based on his meticulous records. He'd also line up all of Mom's prescription bottles and make charts about her dosages. If she began to slip using the new regimen, Dad called her psychiatrist and used his records to challenge the doctor's changes. And many times, if the doctor rebuffed his suggestions, Dad convinced Mom to do what he recommended anyway. "Look, Helen, when you were taking X twice a day, you did fine. Now go back to doing that for a few days and see how you feel. Then we'll tell the doctor."

But no matter what the doctor prescribed or how Dad fiddled around with her medications, Mom had serious bouts of both anger and despair. What I didn't know at the time was that her medications could cause severe mood swings, anxiety, nervousness, confusion, and agitation. So even though we thought that pills were going to magically make Mom better, it's very likely that the combinations she took led to some of her more bizarre and disturbing behavior.

I'd never describe my mother as defiant, but one episode stands out where Mom clearly wanted things her way and wasn't about to yield to Dad in her customary manner. One summer day when I was about eight or nine, all of us were playing in the basement when we heard Mom and Dad shouting at each other upstairs. We huddled together, listening to our parents argue, speaking louder and more angrily with every minute. They never raised their voices to each other, so we were all upset. Afraid of what might happen and feeling protective of my younger siblings, I shepherded them out the basement door and marched them across a four-lane highway to the safety of our aunt's house.

Aunt Emily lifted her eyebrows, and her mouth fell open when she saw all of us bunched together on her porch. I held Kelly's hand and asked if we could come in. As soon as we sat down in her quiet living room, the story about Mom and Dad's fight just poured out of me. She perched on the end of her chair and waited for me to finish, then assured all of us that everything would be fine. She settled us with a snack and then ushered us outside to play on the swing set. She must have called Dad, because a little while later he appeared and told us things at home were fine. He laughed nervously as he explained to Emily that we'd misunderstood what we heard, then piled all of us into the car for a tense ride back home. Dad said something like, "Your mother and I were having a discussion, that's all. Everything's fine," as an attempt to reassure us. The memory of my parents yelling at each other and my instinctive herding of my siblings to a place of protection lived on in my memory for years, and it must have jarred my aunt as well. She brought it up many times over the years.

My sisters described another bizarre incident that occurred several years later, though I must have blocked it out of my mind. They told me that one Sunday morning, Mom stumbled out of her bedroom in a nightgown and marched into the kitchen where she grabbed a few pills from one of the medicine bottles. Instead of taking them like she normally would, she balled them in her fist and headed for the hall closet, looking for her coat.

"Mom, what are you doing? You're not dressed."

"I'm walking to Maple Park."

Maple Park was one of the state mental hospitals several miles from our house. Even as young as we were, we knew about Maple Park. School kids made cruel jokes about the crazy people locked away there. We were all afraid of the place. But we knew, even as bizarre as Mom's behavior was that day, she didn't belong at Maple Park.

None of our pleading affected her—she seemed blinded by some kind of awful pain. Mom charged past us and bolted out the door.

"Call Dad," someone said. One of us raced for the phone while two of us followed Mom outside. Someone tackled her, and she fell to the ground. It took two of us to restrain her. Dad flew home through the mostly empty streets of the city and pulled his car into the driveway. His face was ashen as he approached Mom and helped her up off the ground, looping her arm through his, and guiding her back into the house. He steered her toward the bedroom and locked the door once they were inside. We could hear Mom crying and Dad's reassurances while he talked her down, as he'd done countless times before. He called the doctor for guidance about medication, and he may have taken her to therapy later in the week. Besides the pieces of the story my sisters told me, I have Dad's notation in his medication records for April and May of 1965: "Very agitated...Left home very early Sun. May 30 early AM in (night)gown and overcoat and handful of 1½ grains of NaBut (Nembutal, a barbiturate)[6]."

I've been turning this story over and over in my mind since I heard it. I've closed my eyes and willed myself to remember that Sunday morning, but everything is blank. What was behind Mom's misery, what was so awful that she wanted to escape our house and walk into a state mental hospital? Why did she have such moments of despair? After Dad died, tucked in among old letters and documents, I found some notes from Mom that he'd saved. The ink still looked fresh on the page, and Mom's handwriting was neat and legible. Dad had written the date at the top, May '65, the same month of Mom's Sunday meltdown.

"I have just taken 50 sleeping pills—can't stand it any longer. Somebody must do something for me. Helen."

Clearly, Mom was desperate, and I'm guessing the note preceded the attempted escape. But the note raised more questions than it answered: What did Dad do when he found it? Did he intervene in any way or ask for help from Mom's doctor? Or was Mom taking fifty sleeping pills just one more nightmare in a long string of terrors that Dad endured? Why in the world would Dad have kept such a note and leave it with all of his other papers? I can only guess that he felt it was important enough to save and maybe my witnessing it all these years later is a way of offering comfort to a man who was so desperately alone in his journey.

And what was the doctor's response to Mom's frantic cries for help? I don't see any increase in doctor's visits for therapy; instead, he prescribed a new antidepressant for a few weeks. Dad's margin notes say that the drug made her feel better, so she discontinued it. Boy, do I remember that game. I don't know what her doctors recommended or what the common practice was in the sixties, but Dad stopped and started Mom's medications frequently. If she began to improve, he'd tell her to discontinue taking the pill he decided was responsible. If she worsened, he increased it.

Maybe none of the doctors had explained to Mom and Dad that antidepressants didn't work like aspirin—you can't just take it when you feel bad and stop taking it when you feel better. From what we know now, it's never a good idea to stop an antidepressant cold-turkey because doing so creates all kinds of blowback. Besides the antidepressant, she was taking two kinds of barbiturates and a drug called Miltown for anxiety. Dad used to shake his head over how many pills Mom took and concluded, "She has a high tolerance." It appears that Mom's doctor was very much in the game of giving her lots of drugs to manage her symptoms of depression, anxiety, and sleeplessness. Unfortunately, all of those problems could also have been the result of the drugs she was taking. Dad's final entry for May '65 reads, "She feels the need of Dexamyl, (a combination amphetamine and barbiturate), however, and S. (her psychiatrist) goes along with her."

It was almost impossible for me to believe that all of the pain that Mom endured resulted from having a baby, yet over and over, Dad told us that Mom's condition was due to postpartum depression. No one ever explained her illness to us, so we grew up with the notion that depression was a permanent condition. It became something you lived with that haunted your life, at least that's the way it looked to me. As I got older, I figured that Mom was never able to recover due to her drinking. After all, it seemed like she was doing what was necessary to get out of depression—take pills and go to therapy, but, still, she seemed unable to find her old self and resume a more normal and happy life. I resolved that I'd never be like my mother. I'd do whatever I could to avoid the specter of depression that haunted her for so long. And more importantly, I'd stay away from any of those useless pills she took every day.

Even though I had some thoughts of the possibility of postpartum depression when my husband Randy and I had our son in 1980, I sailed through the experience of being a new mother. Connor was a very easy baby, napping for a solid three hours in the morning and the afternoon and then sleeping through the night at six weeks. I thought the whole baby thing was a breeze and proceeded to take on a part-time job teaching bread-baking and low-calorie cooking for the county extension service. After Connor turned one, I added a part-time job in a retreat center as part of the team working with high school kids. In the fall of 1982, I eagerly anticipated the birth of my second child and believed that I'd continue working after she was born. But I was unprepared for the "new normal" I encountered after Eileen's birth.

Things had started badly right from the moment she arrived. I nursed her too much the first day and woke up the next morning with red, bleeding nipples. Her tiny mouth could barely latch on, and her sucking was so strong I winced every time I had to feed her. Randy was eager for the two of us to come home, so we only stayed one night in the hospital. Eileen developed jaundice the next day, and we had to take her to the pediatrician for an emergency visit.

She nursed every four hours around the clock, and I quickly became exhausted.

When Eileen was one week old, Randy signed up for a Saturday tennis tournament. I woke up groggy, and my body felt unusually warm. My breasts were hard and sore. The pain was nearly unbearable. Could it be a breast infection? A temperature check confirmed my suspicions—it was 103 degrees—no wonder I felt awful. And things were about to get worse when I had to ask Randy for help.

I propped myself up on one elbow and said, "Randy, I'm sick. Can you please take Connor to your mother's for the day? I'll be OK with the baby."

"I have a tournament today. If you can't handle two kids on your own after your mother's been here all week, there must be something wrong with you. Call *your* mother." He headed for the bedroom door then and glared at me.

I fell back into bed and shivered as I pulled the covers up to my chin. "Randy, please, I have a 103-degree temperature and a breast infection. My mom's been here all week. Connor's no trouble. Please, call your mother."

"All right, but I still think you should just take the kids yourself or call Mimi. She's always ready to help." He slammed the bedroom door and went to eat breakfast.

Too sick to fight with him, I called Mimi, my long-time friend who'd introduced me to Randy. I closed my eyes and remembered what I had loved about him when we met. I loved to run my fingers through his shock of long, blond hair and playfully tug on his curly bronze beard. His clear green eyes sparked with mischief as if he were thinking up a new joke. He put people at ease with his corny humor, projecting confidence no matter who was around. I gravitated to Randy because I was shy, and his teasing made me laugh and relax, especially in a group. But over the years, as his teasing and humor became more piercing, often to the point of making me cry, those same traits served to drive us apart.

Thankfully, Mimi agreed to help. "I'll bring you some soup—and you know I love to play with Connor," she said. Not only did Mimi occupy Connor, but she made my lunch, rocked the baby, did laundry, and made dinner so all Randy had to do was heat it up. I slept all day when Eileen didn't need to be fed. But Randy's selfishness didn't go unnoticed by me or my best friend. Mimi tried to be gentle when she criticized him, "Ann, don't you think Randy should've stayed home? Why is he so selfish?" I knew she was right and wished I'd stood up to him, but the fever and aching breasts had held me back.

Deep inside I knew that an even greater deterrent to speaking up and demanding help was the fact that Randy probably would have been nasty to me for days, dropping comments like, "Boy, it's a real shame I had to miss that tennis tournament just because you couldn't handle two kids," or "I guess I'll have to ask permission before I take any time off, right, boss-lady?"

Weeks later when I went in for my six-week postpartum check-up, I told the doctor I was still having after-pains—like menstrual cramps or early labor pains. They were nearly constant and sometimes pretty severe. "I don't remember the cramping being this painful with Connor," I told my doctor.

"Well, sometimes the after-pains are worse with the second child. Give it a few more weeks, then call me if you're no better." He scribbled some notes in my chart and then asked, "What are you doing about birth control?"

"Can you fit me for a diaphragm again? I know they say you need a new one after each child."

After he fit me for the diaphragm and wrote out the prescription, he asked, "Do you want more children?"

I didn't hesitate. "I don't, but my husband hints about another sometimes." I looked down at my hands.

"Why don't you come back with him in a few weeks? We can talk about some kind of permanent birth control for the two of you." He closed my file and sat back in his chair. "Take care of yourself and I'll see you at your next appointment."

After Randy and I met with the doctor and discussed our options for permanent birth control, I had my tubes tied. Eileen was barely two months old. When we'd discussed it before the procedure, all Randy had to say was, "I had hoped we could have a third child, but I guess you can't handle it."

I returned to my former gynecologist because the pelvic pain continued and my OB did nothing to help. When we sat down to talk after the exam, he asked, "How are things going with the new baby?" My eyes flooded with tears.

"I don't know what's wrong with me," I cried. "I'm tired all the time, and I feel totally overwhelmed. My daughter wakes up every four hours all day long, and I feel like I never get a break." My shoulders relaxed a bit.

"Ann, I think you're depressed," he said. "Many women feel that way, especially after the second child." He made a few notes in my file and then looked at me.

My body tensed as anger flooded my system. "I am not depressed," I said. "I'm in pain. What can you do to help me with my pelvic pain?"

The doctor's eyes softened as he said, "I can give you some Tylenol with codeine, but just for a few weeks. If that doesn't eliminate the discomfort, then we'll have to think about exploratory surgery." He scribbled a prescription and pushed it across the desk. "I do hope you feel better soon. Please call me if you need to," he said.

The agony continued unabated for a few more weeks and, eventually, the codeine made me so sick I threw up every time I took a dose. The doctor scheduled exploratory surgery. No pathology. Everything was normal. "Ann, I'm sending you to a neurologist. Maybe there's something subtle that I'm missing."

I was determined to find out what was wrong, why I had so much pain, and then move on and get well. A few weeks later when

I saw the neurologist, he finished his exam, looked me in the eyes and said, "Ann, I think you're depressed." He stood in front of me and waited for my response.

I burst into tears. That diagnosis was the most terrifying of any for me—it meant I could wind up like my mother—depressed forever. I had never known any other kind of depression—to me those words were as good as a death sentence. The neurologist explained how sometimes physical pain can signal depression. "You'll recover," he assured me. "It'll take some therapy, some medication. In a few months, you'll feel much stronger."

I couldn't bring myself to tell anyone that what I was most afraid of was my husband's reaction. I enlisted the gynecologist to tell Randy so that I wouldn't have to face him alone. While we were in the office, Randy acted the part of the supportive, kind husband, but drove home stone-faced and muttered disparaging remarks at me. I remember my stomach wrenching so tightly that I almost gasped at the pain. I bolted from the car as soon as Randy parked.

Things got even worse when I went to see a psychiatrist who prescribed the same antidepressant that my mother was taking—Elavil. Randy was out late on a weeknight—playing tennis—and had been drinking heavily, a continuing and worsening problem throughout our marriage. I sat in an armchair across from the front door, so we saw each other as soon as he walked in. I told him what the doctor said and how I'd need to take meds for a few months, maybe a year, until I stabilized.

"I don't *want* a wife with psychological problems." Randy stood over me and folded his arms across his chest. "I don't *want* a wife who needs to be medicated." Then he walked down the hall and slammed our bedroom door. I wept silently.

Those awful words were like a painful brand of shame on my heart. What kind of wife *did* he want? One like his mother, who bragged that she never got sick? Who always seemed to be on an even keel—but showed little emotion? Determined to be the wife he *would* want, I took the medication only until I felt better, then immediately began to taper it. I had to prove to Randy—and to myself—that I wasn't like my mother—that I could be the kind of wife he wanted me to be. I was strong. I got well. My pelvic pain disappeared, just as the neurologist had predicted. It would take me many more years to realize that Randy's anger served to cover his fear of any kind of illness, one of the "gifts" of his upbringing by parents who boasted about never getting sick.

But Randy's cruel treatment of me when I was in so much physical and emotional pain drove a wedge of mistrust between us. I began shielding myself from him and withdrew in small ways, like going to bed after I knew he was asleep and finding comfort with my friends—people who understood me and built me up rather than tore me down.

Once I was through that period of mysterious pelvic pain and postpartum depression, I had more of an inkling that my mind and my body were sending me messages. But I still didn't understand the language.

Chapter 4: More is Better, But No One Mentioned the Side Effects

Two versions of Mom stand alongside each other in my album of memories: In one version, Mom smiles, puts on a dab of red lipstick, and sails through her days with energy, talking on the phone with her friends and planning snacks for entertaining the book club. In another version, Mom is paralyzed, unable to rouse herself from under the covers, holed up in her bedroom with the curtains drawn in the middle of the afternoon. I never knew which Mom I'd encounter, so I learned shifting roles to fit into her mercurial world. When Mom had her good days, I sensed that she could take care of me, like the other mothers I knew or like my grandmother. I snuggled next to her as she darned socks or watched her as she created beautiful desserts in the kitchen. She often invited me into her room as she dressed and showed me how to wear a silk scarf. They looked perfect on her, but when she offered one to me, I yanked it off, realizing I had many years of growing to do before I could feel comfortable wearing something so sophisticated.

On her bad days we switched roles, and I became the caretaker. I crept into her bedroom and shook her a little, saying, "Mom, come on, you need to get up. I'll help you." If that didn't work, I'd pull her by the arms to a sitting position, then rub her back, making circles over and over. I'd tell her, "Mom, I know you can do this. We'll all help you. Please, just get up and get dressed." Sometimes I actually helped her dress, picking out an outfit for her and then moving her arms and legs through the layers of clothes.

Then, I'd lead her into the kitchen and prepare a small meal. She'd often stop at her pill bottles and dole out her medications, taking them with a gulp of water. When I talked with Dad to get some insight, his explanation for the dark days was standard:

"Your mother had a bad night. She'll be fine in a bit."

Anxiety, agitation, and insomnia plagued my mother regularly and often seemed more difficult for her than depression alone. I remember one day when Mom became extremely edgy, to the point where she behaved more like a drill sergeant than the sweet, soft-spoken woman I knew.

Moira and I were playing house in the basement one summer morning. We each had a wooden doll bed and dresser for the doll clothes—my set was pink and Moira's was blue. Our dolls were seated in chairs at the small table, and we pretended to feed them breakfast. The only noise was the sound of our voices, talking for the dolls, and the chirping of the cicadas in our yard. All of a sudden, my mother clomped down the wooden stairs in her worn saddle shoes and screamed at us, "Clean up this mess!"

"But, Mom, we're feeding our dolls and we've put their clothes away in the dressers," I said.

Mom paced around the room and picked up one of the beds, dumping the blanket and pillow on the floor. "Look at this," she yelled, pointing to the miniature bedclothes.

Moira scurried over to re-make the bed, but Mom grabbed everything from her and said, "I can't take this mess anymore."

Mom turned to me and tried to pull the doll out of my hands. "You're too old to play with dolls."

"Mom, please," I pleaded with her, "I'm only nine." Moira sat in the corner, holding her doll to her chest. Tears streamed down her face. Mom reached for my bed and dresser. I had to act fast.

"We'll clean up, Mom. But please, let us keep our dolls."

I'd never seen her like this, and it seemed ridiculous that she wanted to get rid of our babies. All of our friends played with dolls, and we only had a few outfits for them that we stored in the tiny dresser drawers. I looked around and everything seemed orderly. What was she so upset about?

In the flash of an instant, Mom grabbed the dolls and took the beds with her, clomping back upstairs. Moira and I hugged each other. Then Mom stormed back down the stairs and grabbed the two dressers. "I'm getting rid of these things. It's all too much for me." This time when she went upstairs, we heard the front door slam. We crept up the steps and saw Mom out by the curb, throwing our dolls and their furniture in the trash.

That incident haunted me for years, not just because I grieved for losing my doll and her furniture, but because that day, my mother acted like an alien. The incident never made sense. Until I discovered my father's records about her meds. A quick read of each drug's side effects reveals that alone and in combination with each other, many of the prescriptions Mom took could cause anxiety, agitation, insomnia, confusion, and abnormal thinking.

Even if I didn't know the contents of those amber pill bottles in our kitchen, the culture of the sixties hummed with references to all kinds of drugs—legal and illegal. I remember hearing that Marilyn Monroe had died from an accidental overdose of barbiturates—drugs that calmed you down and made you sleepy, as my parents told me. But no one except Mom and Dad knew we had all kinds of them in our house, a thought which would have deeply troubled me as a child. And while I never directly connected my mother's drowsy state and stumbling walk with the alcohol and drugs she used, I knew the combination was a problem since my parents argued frequently about Mom's drinking and drug use.

As I reached my young teen years and discovered rock and roll on the radio, I sang along with "Mother's Little Helper" by the Rolling Stones. The tune was catchy and the beat was strong. I had no clue the Stones were singing about housewives dependent on Miltown, the first drug used to treat anxiety—a drug that had been sitting on our kitchen counter for years. And when Mom became agitated or anxious, I remember Dad saying, "Helen, go take some Miltown." The phrase "Doctor, please, some more of these" paralleled my father's pleading with Mom's doctor on the phone for more of a certain drug—Miltown or phenobarbital[8]—which he euphemistically called "sleeping pills." But Mom was *sick*, and the medicine she took was to help her get well. That's the way everything was explained to us. In my mind, the women in the song used drugs to escape boredom or tedious lives, as opposed to using them to treat an illness. My mother didn't take them to escape anything, as the song implied. As I watched and listened to all of the adults who came and went from our house, none of them, that I was aware of, ever alluded to Mom having any kind of a drug problem. And Dad? I guess he told himself he had it all under control.

When I started high school in 1966, I couldn't wait to get my hands on *Valley of the Dolls*, a new bestseller about glamorous actresses who self-destructed with alcohol and drugs. The book was everywhere that year, in the hands of kids at the pool as well as their mothers. Of course, the story was tragic, and drove home the point that combining pills and alcohol could result in disaster. But again, I never connected the women's struggles in the novel with my mother's behavior at home. Somehow, even though I talked about the book with my mother, neither of us drew that direct line from the stories in the book to her story. It was as if she couldn't be touched by such an awful fate, since she was under a doctor's care, and the characters in the book were abusing drugs and alcohol—as if the drugs and alcohol could tell the difference. The pieces were all there, but unlike the frayed and fading crazy quilt in the basement, I never stitched the scraps together.

At some point, the chemical load of multiple drugs combined with alcohol was too much for Mom; she began spiraling downward into awful scenes of despair. Back then, doctors still made house-calls—at least ours did. Mom must have had a really "bad spell" as Dad always referred to her dark days, and she was crazy with anxiety. I hated seeing her in that state; she sat on the sofa and breathed deeply and quickly, rubbing her hands in a circular motion, moving in time with her breath, faster and faster, shoulders heaving and brows furrowed.

In looking back through Dad's insurance records about this incident, I'm pretty sure this is the most likely way that events unfolded. Not knowing what else to do, Dad called Dr. T., our family doctor, and asked him to come immediately. Dr. T. arrived with his black doctor's bag, and after a quick kitchen-consult with Dad, talked to Mom and convinced her to come with him. Dad and Dr. T. led her upstairs to one of our bedrooms—probably because it was quieter—and unbeknownst to us at the time, gave her an injection that calmed her down, probably a barbiturate. Emergency handled, or so we thought.

Dad went up to check on her before he went to bed, and knowing how much they were both creatures of habit, he probably gave her the nighttime doses of her pills and supplied her with a decanter of watered-down wine. By that time, we were all accustomed to Dad managing Mom's close calls, so we went to bed thinking everything was fine. But sometime in the middle of the night, a crashing sound woke us up. Moira found Mom at the bottom of the stairs lying in a pool of blood with a huge gash in her forehead and a bone sticking out of her arm. Mom was dazed and slurred her words. Dad rushed out of their bedroom, took one look at Mom, then directed us to clean her up as he got dressed and called the emergency room. We helped her to her feet and draped a coat over her shoulders for the ride to the hospital. She came home with stitches on her forehead and a cast on her arm. I don't know if anyone connected the dots between Dr. T's visit and Mom's fall, but now it seems likely she was seriously over-medicated.

Popular literature also played a part in warning everyone about the dangers of alcohol and barbiturates. One of Dad's favorite news magazines was *U.S. News and World Report*, which ran an article entitled "Battle Against Drugs Turns to Barbiturates." He underlined "Experts warn that barbiturates are especially dangerous when used in combination with alcohol because the effect on the body's central nervous system is multiplied" and "Withdrawal from barbiturates is described by medical authorities as much more dangerous than shaking the heroin habit."[9] But Mom's doctors continued prescribing them for several more years, despite the well-known dangers. And I'm guessing that Dad went along with it, despite his awareness of the hazards, probably thinking it couldn't happen to Mom.

No one openly discussed depression and anxiety when I was growing up, so I was clueless as to why some people struggled with such darkness and others appeared to escape. I knew that I had one tool that seemed to get me through many challenges: willpower. With enough willpower, one could overcome anything, and by the time I was sixteen in 1968, I vowed to never be like my mother. My only doubt about this strategy came wrapped in a warning from Dad who always chided me: "You're too sensitive. Grow a thicker skin." When I pressed him for more of an explanation about causes of Mom's illness, he told me, "Your mother inherited this weakness from her father. He had depression as well." He'd follow that offhand explanation for my mother's deep despair with a caution and a hope: "You want to be more like the Dempseys." That model of inherited weakness from my mother's side and strength from my father's side marked the starting point in my journey to grasp emotional distress.

I had such a limited understanding about the anxiety Mom experienced that I thought it came in only one form—the deep-breathing, hand-wringing version that she exhibited. And while I often felt nervous or worried and sometimes had a lump in my throat, cold hands and churning in my stomach, I never classified those feelings as anxiety. And I had my friend willpower to get me through. I wore the mask of competence, the one role I'd played well for so many years. No matter what went on inside, I maintained a calm and relaxed appearance.

As a teen, one of the most painful experiences I had was the two years of my high school Latin class with Sister L. She stood only about five feet tall, but she carried herself like a giant and rarely smiled. From the first day in her class where she directed us to sit up straight, keep our feet on the floor, and fold our hands on our desks, I was terrified of her. She warned us about misbehaving, telling us, "I taught in a boys' military school, so I know all about bad behavior. I won't tolerate anything but obedience in this room." Sr. L. warned that if we failed to use correct spelling and pronunciation of certain declensions, she'd make us march around the room with a ruler over our heads repeating, "long 'a', long 'a.'"

I still recoil at the thought of sitting in her class for two years, with fear chilling my hands so they felt like I'd been making snowballs without gloves and my stomach churning as if I were being asked to sleep alone in a deserted wood. Sr. L. frequently sent small groups of us to the board for translation exercises where she'd dictate a sentence in either Latin or English, and we'd have to instantaneously translate it. I dreaded my turn at the board. Instead of getting the words in the right order or using the correct endings, I'd mess things up. And when she dressed me down in front of everyone, I'd find myself willing back tears and taking the verbal lashing in silence. Our unit tests consisted of myths written in Latin, followed by comprehension questions and some kind of grammar challenge. My mind would go blank, and all the vocabulary I'd drilled myself on would fly away. I was left with making up the story and answering the questions based on what I could decipher.

One day when Sr. L. handed back our tests, I cringed when I saw a bright red 'C' on my paper. I'd been a strong and consistent A-student all through grammar school, and such a grade stung like I'd been slapped in the face. I kept my head lowered as Sr. L. railed about how stupid our class was. Then she said, "I have three groups in here—the smart group, the middle group, and the dumb group." I kept my head down until I heard her say, "Miss Dempsey," signaling me to lift my face. She finished by pointing her short, arthritic finger at me and pronouncing, "Miss Dempsey, you're in the dumb group."

What I had no way of knowing at the time is that anxiety interferes with learning, that in order to learn, you need to feel relaxed and confident. Fear freezes the brain and renders you nearly incapable of integrating new information. I realize now that my cold hands and churning stomach were classic symptoms of anxiety. It's a wonder I could learn anything in that class, yet despite Sr. L's pronouncement of my place in the dumb group, I had a low B-average for my two years in that particular ring of Dante's Inferno.

I clung to willpower to cope with the frequently uncomfortable feelings. And, certainly, I had been trained to ignore bodily signals in favor of rationalizing. Because so much of my identity was built around being proficient and doing well, criticism from any corner sent me into a tailspin. In my mind, any mistake could result in my friends dropping me or my teachers disliking me. I'd find myself in situations where my body signaled danger, but my mind ignored the warning, especially as I began dating.

My boyfriends were a lot like the men in my family—they teased me and disparaged me over small faults, and then when I got upset, told me I was too sensitive, reassuring me it was all a joke. One of the first guys I dated complimented me on a skirt I'd made by saying, "You're a little chubby, but you're cute." I immediately began the cottage cheese and grapefruit diet to lose ten pounds. When I was a junior in high school, I dated a boy name Will who was a freshman in college. He lived with his mother, a divorcee, who worked a lot of hours. One Saturday, he invited me to his house to listen to a new Rolling Stones album, and I accepted.

"My mom's at work," Will told me when I arrived.

I felt the churning in my stomach, but shook off my parents' strict prohibition to never go to a boy's house if his parents weren't there. I wanted to be cool, so I didn't protest. He fixed us a couple of Cokes, and then said, "My record player's upstairs." More churning in the stomach, but I followed him up the steps to his bedroom. He had the new Rolling Stones album which I'd been dying to hear.

As the music played, we sat side-by-side on his bed and he kissed me. After a few minutes, I felt his hand rest on my waist, and when I didn't move it away, he tugged at my blouse, releasing it from the skirt. His warm fingers brushed my skin and began rubbing my back, inching higher, until he unhooked my bra. We pulled away from kissing and looked at each other—and when I didn't say anything, he began fondling my breasts. I didn't really want him to, but it did feel good and I didn't know how to stop him. *Why didn't the churning feeling go away?* I was afraid if I said no, he'd back out from taking me to the prom. The kissing and fondling went on for what seemed like a long time, until I said I needed to go home. I stood up, turned my back to him, and fixed my clothes so I'd look presentable when I went home. He kissed me at the door and said he'd call later. I hopped in my car and drove myself to confession. *Bless me, Father, for I have sinned. I don't know how to say no.*

Chapter 5: He'll Never Do to Me What He Did to My Mother

In bed listening to my favorite rock music station, WCAO, I wait for sleep. The house is quiet at 11:00 p.m., but I can hear my dad brushing his teeth and using the toilet because we share a wall. Even though I went to bed hours ago, I'm still awake, and I wish I could ask for Dad's help. *What's wrong with me? Why do I feel like I can't learn anything? Why don't I have any friends? Why do I sound so stupid every time I speak?* I wasn't always like this. But now, at fifteen years old and in the middle of my sophomore year, I have landed in a pit and can't escape. I can't feel anything except the ache in my throat that signals a crying spell. I squeeze my arms tighter and burrow deeper into my bed. *No, I can't tell my father. He'll give me those pills he gives to Mom. I'll never let him do that to me.*

Everything seems hopeless, like I'm pretending to be Ann, but the Ann I used to be is nowhere around. I haven't even told my two best friends, Mimi and Carol, how awful I feel. No one would understand. I have to get through it—whatever *it* is—all by myself. Like I've done so many times before.

In my bed in the darkness, I shudder, remembering the time last December when my mother tried to commit suicide. I can hardly talk about it—in fact, no one in my family ever talks about it. But I remember a lot about that night. Like waking up near midnight when my dad yelled, "Ann, get in here!" I ran into the bathroom and saw my mother with blood all over her yellow nightgown, leaning over the sink with her head bowed to her chest. Then I saw the razor on the floor, and I immediately knew what had happened. I'd never seen so much blood. I don't recollect feeling anything, probably because I was so shocked. I reacted instinctively with a first-aid mindset, like I'd been trained to do as a Girl Scout, and immediately tried to stop Mom's bleeding with whatever was handy—towels and washcloths. My mother was white and limp, like a wilted lily. I don't remember her speaking.

At some point, Dad must have directed me to get Mom into their bedroom and have her lie down. Honestly, I don't recall all of the details. What I remember are snapshots—like photographs taken with a flash camera—scenes that stay in my mind.

I heard Dad on the phone talking to someone at the hospital and asking, "Will there be any reporters there?" *What's going on? Why does he care about reporters?* I'm screaming inside my head. *My mother could be dying, and he's asking about journalists!* My brother and sister ran downstairs in response to the noise and found blood all over the tub, the floor, the sink. I was dressing Mom when Dad told me, "I need you to go to the hospital with me." I threw some clothes on while Dad issued a command to my younger siblings, only twelve and thirteen at the time. Neither one of them spoke as they stood in the doorway of the bathroom and surveyed the blood-soaked towels, the stained rug, and the trace-lines of red streaking the tile floor. Moira put her arm around Rory's shoulder as if to support him. "You two need to clean up the bathroom. Just don't let Kelly see this," Dad told them.

Eight-year-old Kelly stood at the bottom of the stairs in her pink flannel pajamas. She wiped the sleep from her eyes and asked, "Where are you going?" while Dad and I ushered Mom out the door. As the door closed behind me, I caught Moira saying to Kelly, "Mom fell and they're taking her to the hospital. Everything will be all right."

I sat in the back of the blue Plymouth and prayed that my mother would be OK. I didn't have my rosary, but I murmured a string of Hail Marys all the way to the hospital. When we got to the ER, a nurse told me to wait in a small, white room; then she wheeled my mother into a cubicle. Dad walked with the nurse, standing guard next to my mother. I was the only person in the waiting room full of black plastic chairs. I stared at the clock and waited, clutching my white corduroy jacket close to my chest. Two swinging doors with small, square windows in them were directly opposite from where I sat. Every so often, a nurse peeked in through the window. Probably to check on me.

But no one spoke a word. No one gave me any news of my mother.

When I caught a glimpse of the nurse, I remember telling myself, *She must think I'm brave because I'm not crying.* Dad came to get me at about 2:00 a.m., and we loaded Mom into the car and drove home in silence. Dad and I dressed Mom in a clean nightgown, and I saw the white bandages binding her wrists. We didn't speak. I kissed both of them goodnight and crawled into bed.

All of us kids got up the next morning, ate breakfast, and went to school. Dad went to work. Did anyone stay home with Mom? I think Dad must have asked my grandmother to come over—I don't remember. I put on my uniform. I went to school. I saw my friends. I didn't tell them anything.

When I got home, I immediately went to the door of my mother's bedroom and knocked softly. She didn't answer, so I pushed open the door. The room was dark. Mom was sleeping soundly, her slender arms at her sides, large bandages covering her wrists. I stroked her short, curly hair neatly arranged on the pillow and kissed her on the cheek. She didn't stir as I lifted her arms one by one and put them under the blanket. I accidentally brushed a finger against the bandage on her left wrist—it sent shivers through my body. I stood in the doorway for a moment before closing the door noiselessly and walking into the kitchen.

I had to talk to someone, so I bolted out the backdoor, charged down the black, iron stairs, ran across the open field behind our house, and knocked on Mimi's door. She must have seen the pain in my eyes and rushed me upstairs. I collapsed on her bed, sobbing into her shoulder. Details of the night before rushed out between my cries. One fifteen-year-old relying on the other in a maelstrom of chaos. Mimi was calm and comforting while facing what must have been shocking news for her as well. I couldn't stay long. I had to get home and make dinner.

The family sat down together at 6:00 p.m., as usual. Mom's place at the table was empty. The dining room was silent except for forks and knives clanking on the plates and some fidgeting in our chairs. At the end of the meal, Dad put his head in his hands and cried. "I never wanted you kids to see this." We'd never seen our father break down. We sat silently. We didn't speak of that night again.

Eventually, Mom's wrists healed. She stopped bandaging them, but the scars were deep and pink. Her doctor put her on some new medicine and changed the dosages, hoping that would help. But after a few weeks when she wasn't any better, Dad took matters into his own hands. Mom usually balked at his choices, but Dad insisted: "Look, Helen, you did a lot better on this combination. Now try this for a few days and you'll feel better." The he put the prescription bottles on the counter, poured a nightly cocktail for her, and she took her pills.

I couldn't understand why Dad didn't tell the doctor about adjusting Mom's drug regimen. We were always taught to tell the truth and accept the consequences, awful as they might be—like a spanking or getting grounded. So why wasn't Dad honest with the doctor? I mean, if the doctor is the specialist and he's supposed to know how to combine remedies to help someone, why was my father interfering? Why did he think he knew better? Why didn't Dad just discuss his ideas with the doctor, share his data, and take Mom in to get her medicines adjusted? As far as I could see, nothing really helped her—not the pills the doctor recommended and certainly not the pills and alcohol that my dad doled out to her day after day. In all likelihood, the doctor never knew about my mother's drinking—not the nightly cocktail, and certainly not the carafe full of wine that accompanied her to bed every night—another thing we didn't talk about.

That fall and winter, I often observed Mom while silently

standing in the living room doorway. *What an awful way to live*, I thought. *I'll never be like my mother.* Meaning I'd never take all of those pills that made her so sleepy, or made her speech slur, or her hands shake. I'd never cut my wrists and try to kill myself.

From what I can recall, Mom failed to get well for longer than a week using any combination of medications. Then she was overtaken by her lethargy and sadness—stopping to rest after cleaning up the kitchen in the morning, crying in her bedroom while she got dressed, cancelling bridge dates with her friends, staying home while I took all of the kids to the library. Descending into her mysterious dark place once again.

Throughout the rest of that fall and into the spring, I moved through my life as best I could, helping my mother around the house, babysitting for my younger siblings, and struggling to keep up with algebra and Latin—my two hardest subjects. And I attempted to get back to some kind of normalcy in my life as a teen. I went out with my friends, attended some mixers at local Catholic churches, and did a lot of babysitting so that I could have spending money. But none of us in the family talked about my mother's suicide attempt. It was as if that blood-soaked bathroom had never existed, even though the scars on my mother's wrists took many months to fade. We did what we'd always done—prayed for her to get better—whatever better looked like. And I vowed to be strong, to be independent. Most of all, to be different from my mother.

And at fifteen, I wasn't like my mother, swallowing copious amounts of Milltown, Elavil, Mellaril, and God-knows-what else. I didn't drink. Not like my mother, who drained a couple of glasses of white or rose wine every night—to help her sleep. But sometimes when I despaired or when I fumed with anger—like when my sister and I fought—I'd find myself in the kitchen pulling Ritz crackers out of the box, smearing them with globs of peanut butter, then eating them as fast as I could. Or taking a custard cup and making a personal-sized helping of frosting, preferably chocolate, and spooning the concentrated sweetness into my mouth, the rich smoothness familiar and exciting on my tongue. Or best of all, making a large, single-serving biscuit out of Bisquick and milk, baking it in a small cast-iron pan and then slathering it with butter. Sometimes, along with my stomach hurting after stuffing myself, great waves of shame engulfed me. I would go into my bedroom, close the door, and get down on my knees. *Please, Mary, I'll never do that again. I hate myself for eating so much. Help me.*

Now, months after Mom's suicide attempt, I'd gained ten pounds. All of my waistbands pinched new rolls of fat. I still hadn't talked to anyone except Mimi about my mother's suicide attempt, or my time at the hospital, waiting alone in that white room. I'd just been going about my teenage life—school, chores, and friends. Now, though, in the darkness, I was in a black hole of pain. But I wasn't going to tell my parents. *Dad will never do to me what he did to my mother. Whatever is wrong with me, I will have to get better alone. There's no other way.*

Chapter 6: Looking for the Why

Dad's records provide more context for what could have driven Mom to attempt suicide. In June of 1967, Dr. S., Mom's psychiatrist, cut Mom's visits to once a month. Dad lists a number of medications that Mom took between May and December of that year, and understanding the effects of the drugs offers a clearer view of how Mom may have been feeling.

The records that I have indicate the prescriptions that were filled between May and December of 1967, so I'm hypothesizing about her condition and basing my conclusions on the effects of Mom's drugs listed beginning in October—Aventyl, Pentobarbital, and possibly Dexamyl. Aventyl, an antidepressant, can possibly cause suicidal thoughts, panic, anxiety, agitation, nervousness, confusion, and nightmares. Pentobarbital, a barbiturate used as a sedative, can sometimes cause anxiety, insomnia, abnormal thinking, and dyskinesia (excessive restlessness), low mood and thoughts of killing yourself, among many other effects. I'm focusing on anxiety and insomnia based on strong memories I have of my mother being extremely anxious and unable to sleep on a regular basis. But while her doctor prescribed pentobarbital to prevent insomnia, he also prescribed Dexamyl—a combination amphetamine and barbiturate—which likely contributed to Mom's sleep problems.[10]

Dexamyl was a combination of two powerful drugs—each used to counteract the other's negative effects. Dextroamphetamine was widely used to treat the symptoms of depression, but it could cause anxiety, agitation, and restlessness, so its effects were modulated by combining it with amobarbital, a barbiturate. A 1963 Smith Kline and French ad for Dexamyl cautions about side effects that include the following: "insomnia, excitability, and increased motor activity."[11]

It's hard to determine if Mom actually experienced suicidal thoughts due to feelings of depression or if the medications themselves caused or exacerbated her already existing despair. Alcohol is the missing ingredient that haunts all of Dad's records, and the effects of alcohol intensified any of the drug reactions.

Some things are just too awful to face—like admitting your wife tried to commit suicide and you had to take her to the hospital ER for care. Dad never talked about that night's horrors, and even in his correspondence, he doesn't reference a suicide attempt. I'm left to wonder if perhaps insurance wouldn't have covered her hospital care if he'd admitted what actually happened. But given the times and the secrecy surrounding all of Mom's experiences with depression, I wouldn't be surprised if he also couldn't bring himself to name what his own wife had tried to do.

Dad saved a note that he wrote to a claims agent regarding the bills for that night and subsequent visits to check on her healing and remove the stitches. There are three sentences in this note that break my heart for what both of my parents endured. Dad wrote: "A female Dr. J. started to suture the lacerations on Mrs. D.'s arms but the task at hand was too involved for her. A Dr. M., apparently the resident surgeon, was called in to do the job. Dr. M. even had me hold her arm while he did the sewing."

Dad had gotten up and gone to work the next day. All of us kids went to school. And that night at dinner, we sat, mutely watching our father cry. All of us paralyzed by the sight of his grief.

And then there was silence. None of us spoke to each other of the event until nearly fifty years later. None of us knew that what we experienced that night was traumatic and could have long-lasting effects. We looked at the suicide attempt as just one more in the awful series of events that happened to our mother that we were not to talk about with anyone—even among ourselves.

Chapter 7: The Long Way Around

Like a persistent shadow that obscures the brightest light, the memories and fears from the night of my mother's suicide attempt plagued me for years. And for much of the time, willpower and competence served as bulwarks protecting me from toppling over an emotional cliff. I considered myself fortunate that since my postpartum experience, I'd been free of depression.

But I hadn't been free from mysterious pain. In the early nineties when I had just turned forty, I had an episode of back pain that hung on despite my best efforts. My family doctor couldn't find anything wrong and suggested I try Tylenol and a heating pad. After a few weeks of following his directions and not getting any relief, I talked with a friend who swore by her chiropractor.

I tried a few sessions with Dr. P., but my whole body tensed when he leaned on me using his full body-weight to push on my back and crack my neck, and I left the office feeling more stressed than when I arrived. After the fourth session, I told him, "I don't feel any better, and I freak out when you push so hard on me. Do you have any other ideas?"

"I think you have pain due to trigger points. Our massage therapist, Hildie, is very skilled in releasing them," he said.

I dreaded the thought of trying another mysterious therapy.

My chin trembled, but I willed back my tears. "OK, if you think she can help me." The aching was wearing me down, and Randy was pushing on me to find a solution.

"You're spending tons of money on doctors and no one can fix you," he said, shaking his head. "This new thing better work." The weight of his unspoken criticism hung on me like a backpack full of books.

I had no idea what trigger points were until Hilde explained the following week: "A trigger point is an irritated knot of muscle that causes pain. I'm going to do some deep tissue massage to release them. Now, take off your blouse and put on this gown, then lie on the massage table so I can get to work."

Hilde's massages were some of the most painful "help" I'd ever experienced. For the first few treatments, I'd lie on my stomach and wince every time she pinched my skin and rolled it between her fingers to release fascia—the layer of tissue just under the skin. I did deep breathing and silently endured what felt more like torture than therapy. "You have many knots," she told me one day. "I'm going to try something new." The next few treatments, she used a wooden knuckle device to go in between my vertebrae and release tension. On the days when I felt better, I thought her treatment could be working. But after about two months of deep tissue work, I continued to struggle nearly every day, so I decided to try acupuncture after a friend recommended her practitioner—Louise.

All I knew at the time about acupuncture was that someone would put needles in me, and the needles could magically help get rid of the aching. But while working with Louise to resolve the physical discomfort, I began learning more about the healing potential of mind-body wisdom.

Louise guided me in understanding some of the metaphorical aspects of my experience. "What could it signify that your back hurts?" she asked me one day. "Think about it after I treat you." For the first time, I considered the intertwining nature of back-pain's relation to my experiences as a mother and a wife, the struggles with my son's spotty school achievement, the increasingly frequent arguments with my husband.

One skillful question can pry open a jammed door, and over the next couple of months, I realized that my back pain was another mask that depression wore. Instead of expressing my emotions by crying or sinking into inertia the way my mother had, my back pounded out distress signals.

Over the next several months, as the pain diminished, relief washed over me the same way it had when I'd taken antidepressants. The sun shone brighter through the trees. The leaves were greener. I felt light and carefree enough to skip down the driveway. Could acupuncture really be as miraculous as an antidepressant? I didn't have any answers, but I knew a good cure when I felt one. In some small way, I'd begun to tap into my bodily wisdom and free myself from pain. For a while.

But my pain holiday ended one afternoon in 1993 when a fierce and sudden headache held me in its grip. I'd had this kind of headache before, several months back, and it went away after a few acupuncture treatments. This time, the pain returned with a brutal energy, and I felt like someone was pouring hot metal over my skull. I looked at the clock: *Two-thirty—I still have time to get rid of it before the kids come home.* But as the minutes ticked by, the pain intensified. I got out of bed and plunged my skull into a sink full of hot water, as long as I could, then pulled my head out and toweled my hair. I heard the kids call out for me, so I put on a smile, gave them a snack, and started making dinner. *Just keep going*, I told myself, *you'll be OK.*

I possessed a lifetime of experience pretending that everything was fine. Going to school the day after my mother tried to commit suicide was my initiation, so after that, I masqueraded as "fine" through many circumstances. But I grew increasingly concerned as the headache hung on for a few weeks, despite acupuncture treatments, Tylenol, and head-soaks. I hid my discomfort from Randy, knowing he'd berate me for being sick and rant about how weak I was. I had to handle the pain on my own, like I'd done so many times before.

When I went to my dentist for a cleaning, I broke down and told him about the headache.

"Maybe you're grinding your teeth," he said. "Try one of those night guards from the sports store and see if that helps."

"Is there anything you can give me to try for a few weeks? I'm completely frazzled by this agony."

"Have you ever tried Valium? Besides calming you down, it can really help with pain," he suggested.

"No, I've always been afraid of it," I said, "but if that could help..." Afraid of it? I was terrified to take Valium, especially after reading the horror story in *I'm Dancing as Fast as I Can* about a female reporter whose life went down the tubes because she got addicted. But I was desperate.

"I'll give you enough for a month. Once you get some relief, you can taper off. I think you'll be fine."

And I was fine within a few days of starting the Valium. Thrilled to finally have some relief, I began tapering after about two weeks of being pain-free. I can't remember if the dentist guided me or if I looked it up in *The Pill Book*—a guide to prescription meds—but even as I went to lower and lower doses of Valium, I remained pain-free. Finally, I stopped completely, confident of banishing the headache for good.

But a few days later as I sat in the back of our friend's car on the way to a new restaurant, twinges of the old headache returned. I brushed them aside, determined to maintain my headache-free state, but as the evening wore on, it became clear that it had decided to return. I cried silently as I lay in bed that night next to Randy and resolved to see Ted, the doctor that my friend had recommended.

After talking with me about my medical history and telling him that Valium had helped the headache until I tapered off, Ted said the weirdest thing: "There's something stuck in your affect, and when it lifts, you'll be fine." Then he wrote me a prescription for Paxil.

I'd never heard the word *affect* before, but didn't want to look foolish, so I played along. Too stunned and confused to ask what he meant, I said, "I've never heard of this drug. Will it help the pain?"

Ted smiled. "Some evidence suggests that this drug can help chronic pain, but it may take a few weeks to work." He continued, "Do you have a therapist you can talk to? That might be helpful as well."

Afraid to find out exactly what he was thinking and why, I grabbed the prescription and headed to the drugstore, hoping for the same relief I'd found with Valium. All of a sudden, it dawned on me. *He thinks I'm depressed.* I clenched and unclenched my fists. *I've done a lot of work over the years and I feel pretty good, except for this killer headache.* My cheeks felt hot and my stomach tightened. *I'll call Fran and make an appointment. I have to talk to someone who knows me.*

After working with Fran for several years primarily on my relationship issues with Randy, I felt very comfortable with her. As I unwound my headache story, I finished by telling her what Ted had said about my affect. I'd looked up the word and understood that it related to the way a person expressed and dealt with emotions. Fran wrote down a few notes as I talked, nodding as I told my story, then said, "I agree that it sounds like you're depressed. Don't you think so?"

As if my posture could mask the panic inside, I sat with my hands folded in my lap, feet tucked to the side, and blinked back tears. "But I've worked so hard on everything," was all I could come up with. *Not this again*, I screamed inside. *What will I tell Randy?*

Fran ignored my distress and calmly told me, "You have a chemical imbalance, and once the meds kick in, you'll be fine. Don't feel like depression is some kind of personal failure." She closed her notepad and tried to reassure me. "Honestly, Ann, if you were a diabetic, would you feel ashamed about taking insulin?"

"Of course not," I said, giving in a little, despite my unwillingness to accept the diagnosis. "I guess I *could* be depressed, but what I'm really concerned about is this awful headache." I wiped a few tears from my eyes. "But how can I be fine one day and depressed the next? Are my brain chemicals that fickle?"

Fran must have looked at the invisible clock on the other side of the room—the one that all therapists have to let them know when a session is over. She stood and began walking me to the door. "Have you read *Listening to Prozac* by Peter Kramer? It will answer all your questions."

Fran and I continued to work together for the next year, but my headache hung on. I found that wrapping a soft ice pack in a scarf and tying it on my head provided a reduction in the pain, so I started wearing that whenever I was home. Randy steamed every time he saw me like that. Paxil hadn't budged the headache, so Ted put me on Elavil for both my affect—now I loved that word!—and my headache. And yes, *Listening to Prozac* told a compelling story about the wonders of the chemical cure for the blues, but niggling away in the corner of my mind, I knew there was more to my depression than some kind of chemical malfunction. If that were the case, why didn't the drugs fix my problems? And why had all those drugs my mother took never fixed her problems? *What if I never got better? What if I really was just like my mother?*

Eventually, after the headache had been around for over a year, I considered the notion of physical depression. I think some people—including doctors—still refer to "physical depression" as hypochondria, and I'm not sure what the actual medical term is, but I do know that in the literature I've read, many doctors reference unexplained physical ailments. Besides experiencing those kinds of ailments myself, I'd seen them happen in my own family—with Mom.

But neither Ted nor Fran gave my explanation any credence. As a general practitioner, Ted had run out of options once we'd tried the standard drugs—Paxil, Elavil, and Serzone. And now, besides the daily headache and the depression, I felt anxious all the time. I decided to give Martin Farmington a call. Surely, as head of psychiatry in our local hospital, he'd know how to help me. I'd admired Martin for years, ever since he'd spoken at a teach-in on my college campus where he recounted his experiences in combat and described how they'd turned him against the war. Because of our shared values, I thought he might be a good fit.

Martin and I worked together for several months, but no matter what medication he offered, my depression hung on. One morning as our appointment came to a close, Martin's voice had an almost sneering tone as he closed my file, then tossed it dismissively onto his desk. "I'm sending you to Hopkins," he said. "They deal with people like you all the time."

"People like me? What do you mean by that?"

Martin crossed his arms. "Look, Ann, you've tried Paxil, Elavil, Serzone, Effexor, Buspar, Valium, and Pamelor—nothing is working. I don't know how to help you, but I think someone at Hopkins can." He smiled, and then made a few more notes in my file. "I'll call them and get the paperwork for you to fill out. It could take a couple of months before you're seen. But they specialize in challenging cases, and you certainly are a challenge." Before I could ask anything else he added, "I'll continue to fill your prescriptions to keep you stable until you see someone at Hopkins. I'm sure they'll get you on the right road."

I didn't want to cry in front of him, but I was feeling less and less hopeful about ever climbing out of this mess. I read books on depression, went to therapy, worked with my prayer group, meditated, exercised—what did I need to do to get better? Martin had encouraged me to talk with Randy about my lingering depression. Up to that point, we'd only discussed the headache, though the longer the pain gripped me, the less strength I had.

"I want you to get better, Ann, but it's a real shame you can't just work with Martin on your depression," Randy said. I sensed that he didn't want to hear how upset I was, so I soft-pedaled the whole issue. Based on his past reactions, I knew I couldn't lean on him.

"I guess Hopkins it is," I said, smiling. But inside I shook with terror. I'd put so much faith in Martin's expertise. *I must be a real mess if someone like Martin is giving up on me.* I continued to push away the thoughts of unending depression, and Martin's callous remarks about "people like me" only served to deepen my resolve.

I knew my depression called for more exploration. And my experiences with other episodes of chronic pain without a discernible cause convinced me that the migraine was related to deeper issues; I just couldn't make the connection. *Here I am, a forty-three-year-old woman with a thirteen-year-old son and a ten-year-old daughter, and I feel like the doctors are writing me off.* The doctors nodded their heads and dismissed me when I said these things, so I turned to books.

When one of the women in my prayer group recommended Thomas Moore's book *Care of the Soul*, I felt like she'd thrown me a lifeline. As I read it, I found words that seemed to be written expressly for me: "What if depression were simply a state of being, neither good nor bad, something the soul does in its own good time and for its own good reasons.[12]" Yes, like the dark night of the soul that St. John talked about. In fact, Moore opens that chapter with a pen and ink drawing illustrating just such a night. The closing words of the chapter buoyed me through many dark months: "We might also discover that depression has its own angel, a guiding spirit whose job it is to carry the soul away to its own remote places where it finds unique insight and enjoys a special vision."

But while I was waiting for that special vision, I needed help managing the pain—physical and emotional. Once Martin referred me to Hopkins, he stopped trying new meds. I was left taking things that weren't working, which made no sense at all. But I continued, because I was too afraid to ask him any questions. Just like Mom. Like straddling a rushing river, I had my feet in two paradigms—one that said depression was the result of wacky brain chemistry and one that said that my soul was working out some kind of mystery, which required patience and faith.

In some ways, the chronic migraines were even harder to live with than depression, but I found some insight in a book called *Paradox and Healing*. The authors, Drs. Greenwood and Nunn, who specialized in the mind-body connection, spoke thoughtfully about the opposing perspectives held by Western medical practitioners and holistic practitioners, and they used stories and myths to explain the mysterious ways the mind speaks through pain.

One story, "The Woman with No Hands," addressed my own struggles. The authors believe that migraines and depression often appear because "…the body is making a stab at communication, but the intellect gets a different message." They view pain that doesn't respond to any medication as a crisis that challenges people to integrate intellect and feelings so that healing can begin and patients can "find [their] own personal power." [13] And while I believed what the authors posit in the book, I still had no idea what was troubling me so deeply that I'd experienced both migraines and depression for nearly two years with no relief. I pinned my hopes for an answer on my visit to Hopkins and prayed.

After nearly two months of filling out forms, transferring my medical records, and requesting an appointment, I sat across from my Hopkins doctor and hoped that he had a magic wand tucked somewhere in his crisp white lab coat. "Bill Phillips—nice to meet you, Mrs. Murphy."

Dr. Phillips scribbled copious notes and asked several questions as I unwound the saga of my history with depression, my mom's illness, and my theory about what I called physical depression. "That's what I think this migraine is about, but I honestly don't know what I need to work on." He flipped through the pages in my file, read something quickly, and then asked, "How did you feel the last time you used Elavil?"

"Like a party girl! I was so happy to finally feel like myself again."

"How long did that last?" he probed.

Though several years had passed, I remembered that Elavil had previously worked almost magically. "Two or three days, then I kind of settled back into more of a routine." I waited as he wrote more notes and flipped through the pages again. "Why do you ask?"

"That's about two or three days too long."

What the heck did that mean? I wondered. *What was he getting at?*

"So, what are you thinking, doctor?"

Dr. Phillips turned in his seat so that he faced me more directly. "Mrs. Murphy, you have mild, atypical hypomania. That means that you have periods of highs and lows, not full bipolar, but still, out of the range of normal emotions."

"What are you talking about?" My stomach dropped as if I'd fallen through a trap door.

"That's probably the reason it's been so difficult to treat your illness," Dr. Phillips continued. "And sometimes, in cases like yours with an underlying vulnerability to hypomania, the drugs can precipitate the disorder."

"Isn't it normal to feel really good for a few days after an eighteen-month depression finally lifts?" *He can't be serious*, I told myself. *He doesn't even know me.*

"Mrs. Murphy, I know this must come as a shock to you, but I want to assure you, you won't be like your mother."

"You're damn right I won't be like my mother. I'm going to get better and won't need all these drugs."

"You will get well—once we find the right cocktail for you. You may need a mood stabilizer at some point, and I'll do my best to find a doctor for you in your area."

I've already been to the best doctor in my area, I thought, *and he sent me to you! Mood stabilizer? Oh, no, there's nothing unstable about my moods. I'm in pain, god-damn it!*

"Wait a minute, please. What do you mean, drugs can precipitate the condition? You mean taking Paxil, Effexor, Serzone, Buspar, Valium, and Elavil—none of which helped me—could cause bipolar disorder?" [14]

"Exactly," he said and turned back to my file to make a few more notes.

"That's absolutely ridiculous. I've never had any signs of bipolar illness—no over-spending, no sexual escapades, no grandiose thinking, no staying up for days. What you're telling me sounds like a side effect *caused* by the drugs, not an actual condition." My hopes slipped away with this new curve ball.

Dr. Phillips sat back in his chair, but before he could answer, I had one more piece of information he needed to hear. "Look, doesn't everyone have a different happiness level?" He looked puzzled, but smiled slightly. I put my hand flat on the table. "If this table is the so-called normal happiness level," he nodded and I continued, raising my hand about six inches above the table, "here's *my* happiness level. I've always been like this."

He looked at his watch and closed my folder, then handed me his business card. "Mrs. Murphy, our time is up. I do hope that you'll feel better soon, once you find the right medication. Call my office tomorrow, and I'll have my secretary give you a few names of people closer to where you live."

Tears pooled in the corners of my eyes, but I blinked them back. No relief once again, after waiting months to see the expert. And what a bullshit story. And now another doctor, more drugs to try. I could barely form the words to offer a perfunctory "Thank you." We shook hands, and I walked down the long hallway to find my car in the garage. I couldn't wait to talk to Fran—surely, she wouldn't go for this line of crap. And what would Randy say? That conversation was shoved out of sight. I couldn't deal with Randy's negativity *and* my own despair.

"I've always thought you were a little hypomanic," Fran said, at my next appointment. "I've never known anyone who's as productive as you, especially when you're struggling with both depression and a migraine."

"So, being a little too happy and being productive are signs of an illness?" Her reasoning made no sense. "You never said anything before, and neither has any doctor over all these years."

Fran launched into a few examples. "You've been very depressed for nearly two years, you have a daily migraine, and yet you still maintain your dressmaking business; you take care of all the household responsibilities, too."

"You need to understand something important. I battle daily with Randy to prove that I'm not like my mother—that I won't be incapacitated by depression. I know I'll get better, and I need to keep my life going to assure Randy and, probably, to assure myself," I folded my arms across my chest. "I'm not doing anything extraordinary. This is me."

Fran sat back in her chair and crossed her legs. "Ann, take a deep breath. I'm trying to help you and so are all of the doctors. Maybe the new diagnosis will help them find the right meds for you. Think positive."

I didn't know how I'd gotten to this place of being called hypomanic, but after a month or so, the idea began to work on me. Maybe I was. I knew I'd always been driven and felt very intense highs as well as profound lows, but never experienced any of the more extreme symptoms. Maybe they were right, but something in the diagnosis didn't seem to fit. My inner voice told me *This is who you are. Happy, sad, thoughtful, intense.* What was it Randy always said to me? "You're so intense I'm surprised you don't wear your friends out."

At some point, I decided it was futile to fight the "Hopkins diagnosis" since once it was in my file, that was pretty much the gold seal of medical opinions. So, I acquiesced to everyone around me and vowed to get better. Whatever pills the new doctor had, I would try. Every day it was harder and harder to feel hopeful. Every day it was more difficult to cope with the unrelenting headache.

I did find a new doctor—a woman—who gained my trust by listening to me in a respectful way. Dr. Wellington was easy to talk to and didn't emphasize the whole hypomanic thing, which comforted me. "Let's keep you on the Serzone, Elavil, and Valium.

I'm switching you to a newer version of Serzone, because I've been getting good results for a lot of patients." I nodded, tired and worn out from trying.

"I'm not feeling as hopeful as before," I told her. "It's been two years and no relief in sight."

"Hold on a bit more, Ann. I know you've had a rough journey."

"Randy and I are going to the Caymans for our anniversary. Maybe I'll feel better after the trip."

"I hope so," Dr. Wellington said. "Be sure and call me as soon as you get home. I'd love to hear all about the islands."

Little did either of us suspect that I'd want to call her *from* the Caymans.

Chapter 8: I Never Thought I'd Do This

Imagine the Dance of Worry and Desire

Imagine a beach
and an amber sun.
Imagine pink crystals of sand
sifting through limp fingers.
Imagine a black lava rock
centered and warm in your palm.

Hear the refrain as rock speaks to arm.
Rub me, arm begs. *Make me bleed.*
Blood the magnet
that pulls you back to life.

Dream that life begs you to stay
for one more dance.
But still you sense nothing except the rock
as it whispers
I can make you feel again.

    The Cayman Islands provided a romantic place for Randy and me to celebrate our twentieth wedding anniversary. One morning we decided to spend a few hours on our own, so Randy set off on a bike ride, and I strolled to the beach. Luxuriating with the feel of fine-grained pink sand between my toes, I stretched out on my towel, lay on my back, and felt the hot sun searing my skin. The waves lapped the shore, making soft whooshing sounds, while the palm trees rustled in the morning breeze. I filled my hand with sand and sifted it through my fingers. I rested a palm-sized lava rock in my hand, noticing how rough and jagged it felt compared to the fine-grained sand. I rubbed the rock on the white underside of my arm and imagined breaking my skin so that it bled. I wanted to feel something, anything—even pain. And if I couldn't feel, I wanted to die.

In 1995, after more than two years of unrelenting depression, my hope was vanishing. No matter what I tried, I couldn't get well. None of the medicines worked. A constant migraine dogged me. I rubbed the rock harder against my arm, then opened my eyes. My arm had bright red streaks on it, but I hadn't broken the skin.

The sun, the blue sky, the palm trees—could my life ever be that beautiful and lush again? Death felt close and comforting, like a rescue boat bobbing off-shore. I sat up and jerked myself back into the moment, pushing away the seduction of suicide. The memory of that awful night forty years before, when my father and I found my mother bent over the bathroom sink, throbbed like a burn that refused to heal. Then I remembered the promise I'd made over and over to never hurt my children the way my mother's attempt had hurt me. No matter how bad I felt, no matter how deep my depression.

Shouldn't I be happy? Here I was in the Caymans with my husband celebrating twenty years of marriage and thinking about committing suicide. What was wrong with me? If I was willing to be transparently honest with myself, I had to admit that my marriage was at least part of the reason I struggled with this tenacious depression. When I was feeling good, I was able to roll with the inevitable periods of bickering and distance, but the longer I felt depressed, the harder it was to keep getting up. The repetitive sound of the waves hitting the shore made me think of all the broken promises and nights of negotiations, and I immediately thought back on an awful argument that Randy and I had had only a couple of weeks before our trip.

Our arguments centered on the trivial, of course, but I knew that was like looking at the tip of the iceberg and thinking if I could only smooth down that ridge, life would be better. Even throughout my darkest days, I'd had to beg and cajole Randy into helping me and showing some measure of understanding. Despite my crushing headache and profound depression, I'd continued doing everything to run the household and take care of the kids. And he'd resisted every time I told him I needed more help—even for small things, like doing the dishes or running one of the kids to a friend's house. Right before we went to bed one night, he told me he wouldn't be around on Saturday, and I burst into tears. "I've just gone through one of the worst weeks of my life, and now you're checking out on Saturday, when I need you."

He propped himself on one elbow and said, "I'm so sorry," then stroked my arm. "What do you want to tell me?"

I sat on the bed, looking down at my hands and began telling him how hard it had been to see a new doctor—yet again—and start another new medication. I waited for him to say something. But all I got in response was snoring. I shot out of bed and headed for the couch. "Wait, Ann, come back and talk to me."

"I just poured my heart out to you and you fell asleep. I don't need that kind of listening."

Randy tried to make up to me the next morning by bringing me a cup of coffee. "Ann, I talked to the kids and told them they need to help you more and not argue about doing chores."

I struggled to stay calm because I'd heard that same sentence countless times. "That's great, Randy, but you need to set a better example yourself. Honestly, most of the time I have to beg you to get what I need."

His conciliatory attitude was short-lived. "If you can't take care of the little bit of stuff you need to do around this place while the kids are gone all day and I take at least one of them somewhere every weekend, then maybe you need to be in the hospital, because

I can't be your nurse."

Every syllable landed like a body-blow. "You're battering me with your words, and I'm leaving." I ran out to the porch and sobbed.

Randy followed me. He knew I was right; I could tell by the softening set of his mouth. "Ann, I honestly will change. I don't want to lose you."

It was as if the dam had broken inside and all the truth I'd been hiding just poured out. I didn't care about protecting him anymore. "All week I've been thinking about committing suicide. Pills, electrocution in the bathtub, or drowning in the quarry. I'm afraid that if this depression doesn't lift soon, no one will want me."

Randy bowed his head.

"I told my doctor yesterday if this new medication doesn't work, I'll get electroconvulsive therapy" (ECT).

Then he hugged me as if to transfuse some of his life energy. "I won't abandon you. Please hold on. We all need you."

The pain coursing through my body at the memory of that argument galvanized me into making a decision I'd long avoided. After two years, no medication had helped me, and facing my days was as arduous as climbing out of a canyon. As I sat on the beach, holding the lava rock in my palm, I knew what I had to do to save my life. In that moment, I decided to try ECT.

For years, I'd avoided the memory of the first time I encountered ECT. My doctors had mentioned that it was done differently than when my mother had been treated in the sixties. But I'd never forgotten that day, and now it all came flooding back to me as I contemplated the treatment for myself.

One evening after I'd finished my homework, Dad knocked on my bedroom door and poked his head inside my room. "You need to meet me after your mother's doctor appointment tomorrow," he told me. "She's having a treatment, and I'll need some help bringing her home." I was sitting at my desk, stacking up my books and making sure I had everything for the next day. Dad handed me the doctor's address written on a slip of paper. "Take the Number 20 bus, get off at Madison, then walk a few blocks to East Chase."

I didn't ask any questions. In my house, if Dad told you to do something, you did it, especially when the direction concerned my mother. Even though Dad was only about five foot eight, he was on the stocky side and carried himself like a boxer.

After school the next day, I got off the bus as directed and walked along the tree-lined streets of Baltimore's Mt. Vernon neighborhood, filled with fading nineteenth century brownstones and brick townhouses. Their wooden-framed windows and cast-iron railings spoke of the city's earlier days. The streets were quiet, despite the hum of cars and buses in the distance. Mt. Vernon had an elegance that even city traffic couldn't disturb.

I found the address easily and walked down the steps to the doctor's basement waiting room. My dad wasn't there yet, so I settled into an upholstered armchair. It was a warm fall day—one of those dazzling Baltimore days when the sky is a bright blue and the trees still cling to their red and gold leaves. The late afternoon sun was giving way to a hint of coolness, signaling evening's approach. I thumbed through a magazine, waiting. No one else was in the room.

Then the office door flew open. Time slowed down as if I were in a dream. I shot up out of the chair, the magazine slipping out of my hands and tumbling to the floor. The doctor and my father each braced one of Mom's limp arms as she stumbled into the waiting room. My mouth dropped open, and a scream stuck in my throat. Her head was bowed and her eyes, normally bright and clear, were mere dark slits. I stood mute, not knowing what to do or say. My stomach churned and my hands went cold. Then both men handed Mom off to me as she slumped down into a chair and tilted forward. I overheard the doctor say, "The treatment went well. She wasn't out for very long. She may be in some pain, though, due to the seizures." *Seizures? Did my mother have epilepsy as well? Why was she practically unconscious? What had this man done to her?*

My mind raced and I choked back tears. I had to take care of Mom and didn't want Dad yelling at me for crying. He thanked the doctor and promised to call him the next day with a progress report. The doctor nodded, then walked back into his office without speaking to either my mother or me. Dad put his hat and overcoat on and walked toward the door of the waiting room.

"I'm going to get the car. Stay here with your mother."

"Mom, can you hear me?" She lifted her head a little and nodded. Still no words. I hugged her and held back my tears.

"I'm here, Mom."

What was going on? Why didn't Dad tell me anything about this place? When Dad returned with the car, the two of us lifted Mom to a standing position and helped her up the stairs.

Once we settled in the car, my mind raced. I thought of Dad thanking the doctor. *Thank him for what?* I wanted to scream at Dad, "What have you done to my mother?" She sat up front, next to him, her head bowed, her voice absent except for an occasional moan. I remembered the doctor saying something about headaches. Sitting in the back of the car, I wrapped my arms tightly around my middle and prayed for a miracle.

When we got home, Dad and I steered Mom into their bedroom where he undressed her and put her to bed. My siblings and I knew what to do. None of us said anything. No questions. Over the years, we'd been conditioned to take care of things—get dinner, do homework. We ate in silence, and then I cleaned up the kitchen. As I dried the last of the dishes, Dad walked in and locked the door, signaling an important conversation was about to take place.

"I want to explain what happened to your mother today," he began. "Come sit at the table so we can talk."

"Your mother was given Electroconvulsive Therapy

treatments—ECT—a few times when she was seriously depressed right after Kelly was born. Do you remember when she was in DeSales Institute?"

I nodded. That was the name of the local, Catholic, psychiatric hospital where my mother had spent about six months in treatment for severe postpartum depression.

Dad said, "Sometimes, ECT was the only thing that helped to snap her out of it."

"How could I forget?" I said. "Mom was gone for months and you never told us where she was."

I caught myself when I saw Dad clenching his jaw. I didn't want to risk his ire and the possible deep-freeze that inevitably followed. Every few months, Dad retreated into a gloomy silence, seemingly for no reason, for three or four days at a time. During those times, everyone—including my mother—became quiet and solicitous. Then, just as mysteriously as the silence had come over Dad, it would depart.

I didn't want that to happen now, so I said, "I understand why you didn't tell us. It was just hard, that's all."

Dad ignored my foray into the past and went on with his explanation. "Dr. Perry is very highly regarded in the community and does a lot of ECT treatments for people like your mother. I'm hoping he can help her."

I nodded. "How do they do an ECT treatment?"

Dad explained the procedure. It was the first time I'd ever heard of electric wires being attached to someone's skull so that they could be deliberately shocked to induce a seizure—something I'd only read about in novels, but I had no clear picture of what one actually looked like. "And because Dr. Perry performs ECT in his office instead of the hospital, he doesn't administer anesthesia. I'm hoping that your mother gets better with this treatment, but she may need more."

Dad and I rarely discussed Mom's ECT after that night, and I do remember that, eventually, Mom improved a little—at least she seemed to surface from the depths that had trapped her. And from the little bits my doctors had told me, all ECT was done in hospitals now, so the awful scenario I'd witnessed with Mom and Dr. Perry wouldn't happen to me. Now I had to get to the other side of this trip and start talking with my doctor—and find a way to tell Randy.

Chapter 9: If It's Not Working, Do More of It

How do we deal with anything that's stuck? Most of the time, the natural inclination is to push harder—an example of "more is better" thinking. And while that approach is sometimes successful, you run the risk of damaging whatever you're forcing. Like people who are experiencing depression.

I found an example of this "more is better" approach in a 1961 article in the *British Medical Journal*. The author discusses the variety of modern treatments for patients with depression who had the vaguely worded "previously good personalities." His list includes the new antidepressants, ECT, long- and short-acting barbiturates, amphetamines, tranquilizers, and modified forms of leucotomy (lobotomy). The author concludes by saying that with all of these modern remedies, few people remain who cannot be helped back to living happily. [15]

I am mystified as to how anyone can think that lobotomies are a good treatment, and by 1961 doctors were well aware of the dangers of barbiturates and amphetamines[16], but it seems that much of the "art" of psychiatry is akin to throwing darts at a target when you're blindfolded. You know there's danger, but hitting the target is also a possibility. Someone may get hurt, but someone may win.

Mom told me several times that the ECT treatments helped her, and Dad used to say they were the only thing that made her better. But according to research, at best, ECT, no matter how it works, only results in a short-term improvement. It doesn't result in a full remission—something that Mom never experienced. Dad saved a 1986 *Wall Street Journal* article that summarizes the limits of ECT this way: "Physicians point out that ECT isn't a cure for mental illness. It's a short-term treatment for conditions that haven't responded to other treatments. Relapses are common…and they really don't know how ECT works." [17]

What kind of person would give such a brutal treatment? That question led me to investigate doctors' attitudes in the 1950s toward using ECT to treat depression. Dr. Sherman, the doctor who eventually administered several rounds of ECT for me, used to say things to me like "I'm going to zap you really good today," and "I really juiced you." Looking back on those remarks, I cringe at the thought of what I was willing to undergo to find my way out of a seemingly interminable depression. Still, I had the sense that my doctor genuinely cared about me and wanted to help me find a way back into the light. The idea that he was on my side possibly helped my eventual recovery.

And my ideas about the value of a trusting relationship with the doctor are confirmed in a 1956 journal article about somatic therapies—that's how the authors referred to ECT and insulin coma shock. The authors focus on how the relationship between the psychiatrist and the patient helps or hinders recovery. [18] And certainly, after seeing four or five psychiatrists, I felt lucky to have someone as caring as Dr. Sherman—someone who was present to my pain.

According to some doctors, insulin coma therapy provided more opportunity for patient-caregiver relationships. This therapy induces an excess of insulin, resulting in convulsions and a coma. Once the patient wakes up, nurses provide patients with lots of attention, such as spoon-feeding, where the nurse acts almost like "…a nursing mother, …feeding him as they do when he is helpless and hungry…as the patient becomes more responsive…a one-to-one relationship with a nurse becomes more effective."[19] The authors portray ECT as a more brutal, hostile, and punishing procedure.

To support this disturbing claim, the authors collected statements, heard many times, made by EST (electroshock therapy or ECT) providers in Britain and the United States over an eight-year period. Doctors and nurses were frequently heard saying things like "Let's give him the works," and "Hit him with all we've got." By far, the most disturbing comment reported came from nurses who suggested "a few shocks" for a patient who "had been fighting, resistive, uncooperative, or obscene in his talk."[20]

The authors conclude by saying that "the success of EST [ECT] …in depression is thus associated with hostile or punishing attitudes on the part of the therapist which corresponds with the impressions received by the patients." The authors trace these harsh attitudes back to the doctors' initial medical school experiences with cadavers, whose passive state becomes the idealized version of a patient for all future contacts.

When I had the ECT between 1995 and 1997, my doctors and nurses told me how safe it was. They assured me that I'd have no lasting memory damage and that any memory loss would most likely be for recent events. I knew that the procedure induced a grand mal seizure, but I was so desperate to stop feeling suicidal that I was willing to do anything. I'm guessing that my mother felt the same way when she decided to see Dr. Perry for treatments.

Although I was driven by intense curiosity to find out what happened to my mother and what doctors most likely believed at the time, I was often sickened by the cruelty I found. Some doctors even believed that memory loss was essential for ECT's effectiveness, such as neurologist and psychiatrist Abraham Meyerson, who said, "I believe there have to be organic changes or organic disturbances in the physiology of the brain for the cure to take place. These people have for the time being more intelligence than they can handle…and the reduction of intelligence is an important factor in the curative process."[21]

Dr. Peter Breggin is one of the most vocal critics of ECT and has long advocated for the FDA to test the safety and efficacy of both ECT machines and the procedure itself. He cites forty-five years of disputes around the safety of ECT and describes years of studies that show ECT "produces enough trauma to the brain to cause a severe grand mal convulsion...and produces symptoms of head injury including severe headache, memory dysfunction, disorientation, confusion, lack of judgment, and unstable mood." Breggin concludes by saying that "controlled clinical trials failed to demonstrate any positive effect beyond four weeks...and repeated attempts to show a reduction in suicide risk have failed."[22]

From everything I've read about the treatment of depression during the time of my mother's illness, each of Mom's doctors was following the standards of the time. And all of the interventions fit into the model that depression was caused by some sort of brain dysfunction that was best treated with medications or brain-altering therapies, like ECT or insulin coma therapy. Some talk therapy was provided of course, but I'm not sure how helpful it was for my mother to talk with her male psychiatrists, especially given the medical establishment and cultural attitudes toward women at the time.

Many in society saw women's anxiety as a result of abandoning their "true, domestic nature," and a 1968 drug company manual, *Aspects of Anxiety*, characterized women this way: "Women, being feminine, are irrational, complaining, and given to tears."[23] According to one researcher, tranquilizers were used to "revive their feminine qualities of submissiveness, nurturance, and familial devotion."[24] It seems to me that doctors believed far more in the power of chemical interventions than they did in the power of human connection, and the long list of my mother's medications is a testament to that way of thinking.

And given that my father never mentioned my mother's drinking patterns, I can only fault the doctors for so much. Would they have continued to give her so many barbiturates, amphetamines, and Thorazine if they had known how much alcohol she consumed? I hope not. But I'm still stuck with the question of why they gave her so many medications when there was clearly knowledge of the dangers of addiction in the case of barbiturates and amphetamines, and of tardive dyskinesia (tics) in the case of Thorazine and all of the major tranquilizers or antipsychotics.

In 1986, Psychiatrist Robert J. Campbell talked about medication's limits for treating depression: "There was a great hope we had found the chemical answer…[but] the anti-depressants don't work for up to a third of depressed patients."[25] Looking for the chemical answer is probably what led Dr. J., one of Mom's psychiatrists, to prescribe Thorazine (major tranquilizer/antipsychotic), Dilantin, (an anti-seizure medication), Dalmane, (a benzodiazepine similar to Valium), Elavil, and Mellaril (an antipsychotic). By any stretch of the imagination, one would think that if the drugs *do* work for two-thirds of the patients with depression, then at least something in that long list would have worked for Mom.

Chapter 10: Getting with the Program

When we got home from the Caymans, I met with Dr. Wellington and told her, face to face, "I felt suicidal and wanted to harm myself—I tried to on the beach with a lava rock." My years of reciting a string of sins in the darkened confessionals of Catholic churches helped me to push through the shame I felt in admitting what I'd wanted to do. I knew that if I couldn't "confess" the shameful things, I couldn't get help.

And I thought it would be as simple as scheduling the procedure and getting on with things. But Dr. Wellington told me that I needed to go to an outpatient facility to be "evaluated" for ECT. "You'll meet the doctor who administers the ECT and participate in an evaluation to determine if it's the right course of action for you," she explained. "The program runs from Monday to Friday."

Oh, God, more waiting? More doctors? I've just told my doctor I want to hurt myself, so why all the delay?

Telling Randy about my decision went better than I'd expected, probably because I'd finally been so brutally graphic about my suicidal thoughts before our trip. I waited until after dinner when he had shaken off the stress of the day. But all of my worry was for nothing when Randy responded supportively and promised to be there for me.

I didn't know what the outpatient program was about, except for making money. Until I walked into the psych ward of South General, I never saw myself as severely ill, but, instead, as someone for whom the routine meds weren't effective. The doctors had another term for it— "treatment resistant."

As I stood at the nurse's station completing my intake form, I got a look at some of the other patients. One woman was catatonic. She shuffled down the hall, gazing ahead with a vacant stare. Her speech was unintelligible. Another woman wearing a nondescript sweat suit pushed her unkempt hair out of her eyes. She stood next to me and held herself in a stooped posture, rocking back and forth as if she were sleeping. A twenty-something man danced down the hallway and made nonsensical remarks to the nurse. *I don't belong here.*

But the nurses acted like everything happening around them was normal. Felicity, the nurse assigned to me, interviewed me and then explained the schedule for the week.

"First, you'll have cognitive therapy, then you must attend a drug and alcohol abuse education session; lunch follows—you have thirty minutes to eat—then you'll go to occupational therapy for an evaluation. Tomorrow will be the same schedule, but you'll have a feelings group instead of cognitive therapy." Her crisp British accent made the schedule sound even more boring and onerous.

Hmmm, just like Catholic school. There is only one way to go, no exceptions. I know how to do this. Just say yes to everything, get the ECT, and get out of here. "Sounds like a plan," I said. She smiled and led me to the next stop on the evaluation train.

I made it through cognitive therapy where we talked about how we could change our negative thoughts to positive ones— which I had already been doing for a year or so. I was confused— was I in a new therapy group or were they evaluating me on the sly using the cognitive therapy group? But the morning was only halfway over. Next, I suffered through a movie on drug and alcohol addiction. Lunch was awful—then on to occupational therapy.

My evaluation with Bonnie, the OT, consisted of threading a leather lace into a square piece of cardboard with holes punched all around its perimeter.

I've been sewing all of my own clothes for the past thirty years. This must be a joke. I wanted to grab the stuff out of her hands and throw it on the floor. Ever mindful that I was being evaluated and compliance was highly prized in a psych ward, I smiled and did three stitches, up and down, but managed to twist the leather since it was worn and thin.

"Does yours look like mine?" Bonnie shook her head as if she had to give me the answer. "I'm going to let you try it once more." She handed me the square.

Hold back, Ann. If you scream at her, she might think you're belligerent or combative.

"Oh, I see now," I said in my most obedient, Catholic-girl voice.

When I finished the three stitches—perfect this time—Bonnie chirped, "That's wonderful! You showed very little anxiety." *Why would I?* I smiled at Bonnie and looked at the clock. *Day one is almost over. Twenty more minutes and I'm out of here.*

On day two, I attended a "Feelings Group" with a therapist named Valerie. After all of the participants agreed to maintain confidentiality, several people spoke about a variety of difficult life situations. Then I jumped in.

"I'm *feeling* angry and frustrated with the whole healthcare system. I've had ten doctors and/or therapists in just over a year and now I have to deal with two doctors here—one for my meds and one for the ECT. The new psychiatrist at my HMO seems helpful and caring, but she sees patients all day long—for fifteen minutes each."

My words had awakened everyone, and the room pulsed with more angry voices. Everyone had a story to tell about the ravages of "the greatest healthcare system in the world," and poor

Valerie struggled to regain control of the group. "Keep with the feelings," she reminded us.

Several of us replied together, as if we had a script, "Anger, rage, and frustration *are* feelings."

Valerie demonstrated clearly that she'd been schooled in the ways of the system when she asked, "Have any of you joined the Alliance for the Mentally Ill? They work with state legislatures to pass laws for more favorable treatment for people like you." *People like you? Damn, and she's a therapist?* Clearly, she didn't connect with our feelings of disempowerment from being handed around from doctor to doctor and prescribed pill after pill. A guy in the corner who'd been quiet during all of the turmoil spoke up.

"Good luck seeing a doctor today, Ann. I've been here for five days and I ain't seen no doctor yet." He leaned back in his chair and propped his legs on the windowsill.

I couldn't hold back any more. "I'm desperate. For the past two years, I've been depressed and had a continuous migraine. Do I have to *hurt myself* before I get to see a doctor?"

The room was silent. Valerie looked at the papers in her lap, then managed to say, "Why don't we end the group here? I think everyone could use a break."

As we filed out of the therapy room, walking as if on an assembly line, Felicity grabbed my arm and steered me into a room where they were just starting the film on ECT. "I'll sit with you and we can watch it together. You'll feel better after you see the film."

The procedure depicted in the film wasn't as bad as I'd feared; there were no patients screaming in agony and rising off the gurney à la *One Flew Over the Cuckoo's Nest*, but the movie had a surreal tone. The voiceover lacked any notes of empathy or support and showed no connection to the painful experiences of people with unrelenting depression. By now, I had experienced many instances of coldness and sterility from nurses, doctors, and therapists working within the framework of the medical model—which amounted to assisting people with chemical imbalances to get their neurotransmitters firing properly again. The medical model assumes that the rest of our lives, with all of the trauma and challenges, despair and loneliness, have no bearing on our feelings of depression and anxiety.

One of the women in the room said she had benefitted from her ECT treatments, then added a caveat, "Some people get better after one treatment, but I need medication and a few tune-ups every year just to keep myself healthy." *Tune-ups? Was she talking about a car engine or her precious mind?* I prayed that I would never need "tune-ups" of that sort. But after consuming numerous medications with no relief, I was resigned to trying ECT and prayed that I'd be one of those people that only needed one treatment.

Later in the day when I once again asked to meet Dr. Sherman—the doctor who would perform the ECT—the nurses told me that he was too busy, but I'd meet him before the procedure. And I'd have another doctor—Dr. Miller—to deal with my new medications. I balked about the clumsy arrangement, but Felicity pulled me up short when she said, "Ann, this is an outpatient facility. You won't have the same doctor all the time."

When I finally met Dr. Miller, he told me, "You're not really out of options, you just think you are. We have many more drugs you can try." *Right. That's why I'm here. Nothing is working, so I'm trying something new.*

He launched into a long description of the two procedures that were available for ECT: "The standard treatment for ECT is to give the patient one anesthesia for each procedure. We'd give you several treatments per week over the next few weeks for a total of up to eight or twelve treatments. We also offer two courses of anesthesia with two shocks per procedure for a total of eight shocks in two days." We briefly discussed the pros and cons of each treatment and then he concluded, "You can go do some research and decide how you want to proceed." *Great*, I thought. *I guess I'll just go to the medical library for a few days while I gather information, interview a few patients, and decide what is best for me.*

The day before my ECT procedure, Felicity announced that

Dr. Sherman would see me—in the hallway. *So much for privacy rights.* Dr. Sherman wore rumpled khaki pants and an Oxford cloth shirt with the sleeves rolled up, and his wiry, gray hair stuck out all over his head. His glasses perched so far down his nose they nearly slid off.

Am I'm going to let this wreck of a man run electricity through my brain? My unequivocal *yes* was a measure of utter desperation coupled with my fierce determination to live.

But Dr. Sherman turned out to be both compassionate and funny, which helped calm my nerves. He loved The Grateful Dead and reminded me of hippie musicians with his ponytail hair and rimless glasses.

"Many of my patients have excellent results," he explained, "meaning that they got out of depression. I usually administer four shocks with one anesthesia."

"Fine with me," I said, relieved that I wouldn't have to gear up emotionally to undergo four visits to the hospital, four times of lying on the operating table, and four separate procedures.

When I had met with Dr. Miller, he'd told me, "The day before the procedure, stop taking your depression meds—Serzone, Elavil, and Valium—so that you'll have better seizures." *Oh, God. I never thought I'd actually want to have good seizures.* I dutifully complied and figured Dr. Sherman would give me instructions as to when to start the meds again. When Randy and I arrived at the hospital early the next morning, I was very nervous and tried hard to be positive about the outcome of the treatment. It was a big step for me, even though ECT happened all the time in the hospital.

As the nurses prepped me by getting all of my vitals and helping me to change into a hospital gown, bonnet, and booties, one nurse, Maggie, surprised me when she said, "You poor thing. You're Dr. Sherman's patient."

"What do you mean? He seems very nice, and he said he gets good results for his patients."

Maggie laughed and winked at the other nurse in the room.

"You know that Dr. Sherman is rather stout—well, last week we were all out of large scrubs, so he wore small ones and his pants fell down in the OR."

"But we made him a pair of suspenders, so he should be fine today."

This comment set me on edge. Before I had a chance to say anything, a new nurse wheeled me into the OR. Dr. Sherman—sans suspenders, so I figured he had the right size scrubs—and an anesthesiologist I had never met laughed and joked while loud rock music boomed, nearly drowning out their voices. I remember the nurse wrapping my left leg with a tourniquet so Dr. Sherman could monitor the seizure by watching my big toe wiggle. So far, it was all just like the film I'd watched. Still, I was extremely nervous and the casual atmosphere in the OR did not allay my fears. When the anesthesiologist finally began talking to me, I begged him, "Put me out, please. I can't take the waiting."

When I woke up, I cried.

Dr. Sherman came to see me later in the recovery room and gave me his view of the procedure. "I gave you four good shocks and you had great seizures. I think you'll see some progress after this treatment. Enjoy your Memorial Day weekend."

But the medical miracle of outpatient treatment still had a few glitches when it came to covering all aspects of my care. I felt nauseated and agitated for about three days after the treatment. Things were so bad that I went to a bookstore to look up the effects of suddenly discontinuing Serzone, Valium and Elavil; I was suffering withdrawal. Since no one had told me to restart my meds, I panicked and called Dr. Sherman repeatedly over the holiday weekend, leaving messages with his answering service. He finally got back to me on Tuesday.

"I'm not in charge of your medication. Dr. Miller and Dana, his physician's assistant, are supposed to handle that."

"I never heard from him after the treatment, and I don't have his number. I've been sick all weekend, and I think it's from stopping my meds cold-turkey, which probably never should have happened. Now what do I do, since I have you on the phone?"

Dr. Sherman started me back on my meds, and upped my dosage of Serzone. I was desperate enough to agree to his direction and even desperate enough to schedule another treatment.

I had a total of seven treatments with four shocks each. Every time I went back, I had the same fears, but at least I no longer cried when I woke up. I did lose chunks of my memory—forgetting that we had purchased a painting in the living room, losing my way to the neighborhood grocery store, asking my daughter where she got her new shoes that we had bought the week before. I'd take copious notes and write long passages in my journal for days before every treatment, never sure of what pieces of my life I might lose.

I still have lots of black holes in my memory, especially for anything that happened in that time span, and I'm always embarrassed and sad when I can't remember what others insist I *must* know. But the things that I'm able to recall are the things that have great emotional weight and importance—like the endless visits to doctors and the ridiculous therapy groups at the day treatment center. And I have the journal that I kept from 1993 to 1997 that contains all of the main events of the time as well as my thoughts about what I was going through.

Even though my hospital experiences were nothing like my mother's traumatic office visits to Dr. Perry, my experience of depression seemed to be as relentless and resistant to traditional treatments as hers. And despite Dr. Sherman's complete faith in the power of ECT to knock out depression, my black mood hung on.

Chapter 11: ECT—the Backstory

A couple of years ago, I found thirty years' worth of my dad's records about my mother's illness. A half-sheet of paper on top of the pile listed the dates of Mom's ECT treatments in Dr. Perry's office from 1968 to1970. She had thirty-seven treatments in a two-year period, sometimes as many as seven in a month. Remembering how Mom looked the day I helped to bring her home, I felt both sickened and enraged when I saw the numbers. I began reading as much as I could find about how ECT is administered and exactly what happens, especially without anesthesia. And for that picture, all I had to do was flash back to watching Jack Nicholson rise off the table screaming in terror in *One Flew Over the Cuckoo's Nest*. When I watched it in 1975, I made a vague connection to my mother's experience and felt extremely disturbed by what happened to Nicholson's character. I think my inability to connect more fully was my psyche's way of protecting me, even seven years after my mother's "treatment."

What happens during an ECT procedure? I'm not sure how much of this information was in the film I watched in the hospital, mainly because the film emphasized making people comfortable with the "procedure." Despite the bland reassurances stated in both the film and much of the pro-ECT literature I've since reviewed, I felt quite disturbed when I did some reading about the procedure itself and what happens in the brain. Doctors usually attach electrodes on both sides of the skull for bilateral treatments, although some doctors give unilateral treatments. Now, nearly all ECT is performed under general anesthesia, and patients are given muscle relaxants. After attaching electrodes to the sides of the skull, the doctor administers 100 to 190 volts of electricity, enough to induce a grand mal seizure and convulsions. The convulsions can be strong enough to cause broken bones, especially ribs, which is why powerful muscle relaxants are needed.[26] Additionally, the anesthesiologist administers oxygen during the procedure because the muscle relaxants often make normal breathing impossible. One effect of general anesthesia combined with muscle relaxants is that it "raises the seizure threshold necessitating a current of greater intensity."[27] One professor who has done extensive research on ECT has found that it's primarily used on women and frequently induces brain trauma, memory loss, confusion, and a sort of passivity.[28]

Up until several years ago, I had complete faith in Dr. Sherman's assurances that ECT was safe and effective, despite his admission that no one really knows how it works. After reading a lot of research on ECT, I felt lucky that I was all right and hadn't suffered more memory loss than I did. While I usually picked up where I'd left off in my life after a treatment, I do recall that after one treatment, I slept almost continuously for at least a week, getting up briefly to see my kids off to camp in the morning and to make dinner in the evening. There's some research to indicate that excessive sleeping after ECT can be a sign of traumatic brain injury, but I have no lingering symptoms. I'm also extremely fortunate that I never had any cardiovascular or lung problems, as happen with some patients who've had the procedure. And you have to dig pretty deep to find out that strokes are also a possible effect of ECT, though the medical literature uses the technical and less layperson-friendly wording "cerebrovascular event."

From what I could find, ECT is always administered with anesthesia in the United States now, but "direct ECT" (without anesthesia) is still practiced in India. According to one journal article I found, a number of doctors there find the practice unethical.[29] I didn't need any convincing on that point. But what was useful for me to discover was the researcher's depiction of how many people are needed to conduct the procedure without general anesthesia. He says that such a team consists of several orderlies, nurses, and psychiatrists—all needed to restrain and protect the patient from harm due to convulsions and seizures.

And after reading his description of the team, I'm left wondering if Dr. Perry had a cohort of assistants to help him or if he used some kind of short-acting sedative, probably a barbiturate, on his patients. I think that my brain is protecting me, because even though Dad said that I went with him several times, I remember only one visit to Dr. Perry's deserted office. Still, he must have had at least a nurse there, based on what I've read.

In one of Dad's letters to Dr. J. in June of 1970, Dad says, "Mrs. Dempsey hates the thought of these treatments, but, actually, she doesn't even know she's had one a half an hour after it's over. Dr. Perry has a unique technique for administering his treatment." I can't imagine that my mother could have endured thirty-seven shock treatments without any anesthesia. I don't think Mom would have cooperated, and I can't imagine that Dad would have put her though such torture.

From reading this 1969 letter that Dad wrote to the insurance company regarding reimbursement for Dr. Perry's billing, it seems that even he was well aware of the bad reputation and negative connotations around ECT:

> *Dr. Perry is averse to calling his "Treatment" Electroshock Therapy as he figures it is upsetting to the patient and their family. Consequently, his bills are marked "Treatment."*
>
> *On the first several bills received from him, when I went to pay them, I requested his secretary to type in "Electroshock Therapy." On his later bills, I just sent him a check and didn't have him add on to the wording of his bills.*
>
> *On all the bills, the word "Treatment" denotes Electroshock Therapy. This can be readily verified by a call to his office. M. T. Dempsey Jr.*

The thought of my mother enduring thirty-seven ECT treatments with minimal anesthesia sickens and angers me. I remember how awful she looked the one time I went with Dad to pick her up, and I also remember her terrible memory losses for all kinds of things. I have no idea if the treatments helped Mom's depression, but the process seems to fall into the category of "if it's not working, we've got to do *more* of it and *push harder.*"

And despite Mom's thirty-seven ECT treatments with Dr. Perry, nothing helped for long—except when she would later be hospitalized and detoxed from alcohol. But Mom could never maintain her sobriety once she returned home to the same routines and pressures. And nearly fifty years later, all I can conclude is that my mother was desperate to live. What else could have driven her to accept such a drastic, traumatic, painful remedy? What must my father have felt seeing her nearly catatonic after each treatment? These are questions I can never fully answer. I'm saving them for the other side.

Chapter 12: Down the Rabbit Hole Looking for Relief

By early 1996, I'd been working with Dr. Sherman for several months, trying to get the depression under control using a combination of psych drugs and ECT. One day we were talking about the migraine—I'd had it every day for the past three years, and the relentless pain complicated every level of my attempt at recovery.

"I know this headache is stress related," I told him, "but I'm not sure what I'm stressed about."

"Even if your headache is stress related, you need to see a neurologist to rule out any organic issues," Dr. Sherman said, and then scribbled the name of a doctor for me.

"I'll go if you think I should, but I've been through this scenario before—having serious physical pain with no obvious cause. I call it physical depression, but I'm sure there's a medical term for it." I tried one last time: "I've told you about the other times I had chronic pain and it was actually a form of depression. I know the headache is from stress."

As Dr. Sherman scribbled a referral for me, I thought back to 1973 when I was a junior in college and my mother struggled with debilitating tooth pain. She visited numerous dentists, hoping one of them could uncover the source of her distress. But most days, Mom spent hours sitting on the worn, brocade sofa with her left arm propped on a pillow and her hand holding a heating pad to her face. One evening, I overheard Dad talking to someone on the phone, describing Mom's plight.

"Yes, Helen has a mysterious toothache and she's been to four doctors. One of them suggested that she have all of her teeth pulled."

Mom rested on the sofa, in earshot of Dad's conversation, with a blank look on her face, her hazel eyes pale and downcast. No matter what kind of pain she was experiencing, she seemed determined to stay up until 11:00 p.m., her arbitrary bedtime. Dad continued, "Finally, her psychiatrist intervened. He thinks the pain is a form of depression and suggested a new medication as well as hospitalization."

Mom spent the next several weeks in the psychiatric ward of a local Catholic hospital. We weren't allowed to visit her for two weeks, and, of course, no one gave us a reason. Just recently, my brother Rory told me that Mom's doctor thought she was severely overmedicated and he needed to detox her—which is why we weren't allowed to visit. I didn't know about Mom being detoxed at the time, but maybe Dad had confided in Rory since they were so close. When the doctor felt that Mom had stabilized, I remember visiting her and noticing how much happier she seemed, how alert she was. "I drink a cup of warm milk before bed," she told me, "and it actually helps me relax."

Once she got rid of the toothache and went through detox, Mom was the best I'd ever seen her. Based on Mom's results, it seems obvious that the doctor made the right call for her when he recognized her intense physical pain as a sign of depression. Here's a letter that Dad wrote to one of the sisters who had worked to get my mother admitted to the hospital:

```
March 25, 1974
Dear Sister Paulette,
     A year ago, my wife was a patient at St.
T.'s and I feel it was only through your
understanding of her problem that she was
```

> admitted. Prior to this she had run the gauntlet of specialists and none of them knew what she needed. I was almost at the point of dropping her on the doorstep of a hospital and say[ing] she is really ill, take care of her.
>
> I am very happy to report that the past year has been the best year she has had during the past sixteen years. Our four youngest children, ages 15 to 21, have never seen their mother so lively and vibrant as during the past year. They are amazed at how she has been. All they ever knew was a sick mother.
>
> Again I want to thank you for what you made possible. My heartfelt thanks to you.
>
> Cordially, MJD Jr.

When Mom first came home, she continued drinking warm milk instead of wine, but she couldn't maintain her sobriety. I'm guessing Mom had a lot of support for her healthier habits in the hospital, but since no one got the family on board with her healthier habits, Mom eventually slipped into her former practice of drinking wine at bedtime. Over time, the depression crept back in, but, thankfully, the toothache was gone for good.

I reminded Dr. Sherman about all of my experiences with mysterious pain and even threw in a few details of what my mother experienced, but he stuck firmly to his opinion.

"Go see my friend, then we can talk again."

I think every other doctor had been willing to believe me as long as I wasn't banging the door down demanding an end to the pain. Maybe Dr. Sherman was right about sending me to a neurologist. And I was too tired to fight with him.

I saw the neurologist a few weeks later—he couldn't find anything that might cause my migraine. Family history of migraines? No. Problems with light and food triggers? No. Headaches related to my cycle? No again. The neurologist flipped through my records one last time, rubbed the bridge of his nose, then took off his glasses and cleaned the lenses. He was as puzzled as all of the other doctors I'd seen. "I can't find anything wrong with you, but since you're obviously in a lot of pain, check out Dr. Mitchell's headache clinic. They help lots of folks and use cutting-edge research in their treatments." He handed me a card with the information and sent me on my way.

It was weeks before I finally got an appointment at the headache clinic. When I finally met with Doreen O'Neil, the nurse practitioner who interviewed and screened new patients, she was very kind but just as puzzled as all of the other medical folks. "Valium's the only medicine that has helped you? Which doctor first prescribed that?" Doreen brushed back her blond hair and waited for my answer.

"I'm not proud of this," I told her, "but I asked my dentist for it." I looked down at the floor and continued. "I was in horrific pain and didn't dare tell my husband, because he always yells at me when I get sick. I went to the dentist for a cleaning and mentioned my headache. He prescribed Valium for me."

My story must not have been that odd. "Go on, then what?" Doreen waited to take more notes.

"After I took it for about a week, the pain was much less. I took it for another week, just to be sure that the pain was gone, and then I began to taper off."

"How much were you taking, Ann?"

"I think I took two milligrams, three or four times a day. The pain seemed to be gone, so I stopped taking it after a few weeks, but about a day or so after the last pill, the headache was worse than ever."

"Do any of the other medicines help? I see here in your records that you're taking Elavil, Wellbutrin, and Valium. Still no pain relief?"

I shook my head. "No, and I'm really afraid. I've had several ECT treatments and I'm still depressed, and the headache pain is awful. I can't go on like this."

"Ann, we have lots of medicines for you to try, and we have good success treating our patients. I'm sure we can help you."

Doreen gave me a physical and then wrote me a few prescriptions—one was for a nasal spray, one was for Prednisone to decrease inflammation, and the other was a new drug that I'd never heard of. "What's MS-Contin? Can I take it safely with all of the other pills I'm on?"

Doreen assured me that I could. "MS-Contin is very safe, and it's not addictive. The studies show that it offers fast pain relief, and many of my patients are doing well on the drug.[30] I'll call Dr. Sherman and update him on the drugs that I'm prescribing. I think you'll feel better in no time." Only years later did I learn that MS-Contin was actually powdered morphine. If I had known then, I'm sure I'd have been terrified to use it.

Doreen's confidence, along with the new prescriptions in my purse, seemed like one more shot in the dark. I walked out of her office and drove straight to my pharmacy. I was almost afraid to hope for pain relief. Doctors had made so many promises—always assuring me that whatever drug I was on would be the one to work. Still, I felt a spark of hope with the nasal spray and the MS-Contin. I'd have to read up on that one. *If I can get rid of the physical pain*, I thought, *I can find a way out of depression. I've done it before.*

I saw Dr. Sherman six weeks later for my regular visit. "How's your headache?" he asked. He smiled as if he already knew my answer.

But my smile served as a mask that I knew I could drop once he closed his office door. As soon as I sat down, I burst into tears.

"I feel like a chemical waste dump," I sobbed. "You have me on Elavil, Wellbutrin, and Valium, plus I've had three ECT treatments, and I'm still depressed. Now the headache clinic gave me Prednisone for ten days, some kind of nasal spray, and MS-Contin. I'm barely getting any pain relief and still need to wear an ice pack all day—except when Randy's around. I'm afraid of what all of these drugs are doing to me."

Dr. Sherman sat in his armchair and wrote down some notes. Then he looked at me, glasses perched on the end of his nose, khaki-clad legs stretched out in front of him. "What do you want me to do, Ann? Sometimes treatments take a while to work. You've got to hang on."

"I'm sick of being told to hang on. I've been hanging on for three years now. I'm in constant physical pain. My depression is just as bad as it was a few months ago. No progress despite all of the pills, all of the ECT. My husband yells at me when I wear an icepack on my head to get any relief. My kids are worried. I'm hanging on, but I'm afraid."

Dr. Sherman was quiet for a few minutes, then he said, "I think I'll put you on some Depakote. You're agitated and sometimes when I add Depakote, my patients respond better to the antidepressants. Besides, even after you stop the Prednisone, some people become manic, and you don't want to risk that with your tendency toward hypomania."

And so it went—he added a new drug, tweaked my dosages, and then scheduled me for another ECT. Doreen finally put me in the hospital to break the cycle of the migraine and while I was there, they pumped me full of IV Prednisone and switched from MS-Contin to OxyContin.[31] I felt a little better when I was in the hospital, but Randy refused to visit me. "I can't stand seeing you in the hospital. Besides, I have to run my business, and I have appointments every night to line up more jobs. Plus, I'm taking care of the kids."

I experienced some pain relief in the hospital, but it vanished within days of resuming my duties at home. Randy never understood that I needed some time to readjust and ease back into my routine. "You've been lying around in a hospital for five days doing nothing while I've been here working and taking care of the kids and the house," he'd say and then storm up to his office for a few hours.

Nearly a year had passed since the last hospitalization, and now the migraine was so unbearable that Doreen decided on a more radical method of pain relief. "Ann, I'm going to hospitalize you again, and this time I'll send you home with a new medication that could help you kick the pain. The only downside is, you'll need to inject it into your thighs."

I burst into tears. "How will I tell Randy? He already yells at me for all of the pills I'm taking and makes me hide them in a cookie tin in the bathroom. He says seeing all of those pills reminds him of my mother."

Doreen nodded. "Why don't you ask Randy to come in and talk to me while you're in the hospital? It sounds like you could use some help getting him on board with your treatment."

"He won't come. He says all of the doctors say I'll get better, but nothing works. He tells me all the time that I'll always be this way." I sobbed and put my head in my hands. "I know I'll get better. I have to believe that. No one stays depressed or has a headache forever."

Doreen came around from behind her desk and gave me a hug. "I have faith that you'll get well, and I know how frustrated you must be. But I've seen lots of patients do well with pain control once we start the injections."

I know that she meant to comfort me, but I was tired of hearing the empty promises every doctor made. Did they honestly know what they were doing? And how could I possibly add one more drug to the list? As I drove home, I ticked them off in my head: for the depression—Wellbutrin and Depakote. Elavil—for both depression and pain relief. Valium for anxiety. Then nasal spray, OxyContin, and now I'd add some kind of injectable drug.

Every time I got a new drug, I'd ask both doctors if they were sure that the combinations were safe. Both of them assured me that what I was taking was fine. But I felt numb. "I can't feel," I'd tell them. "I just want to feel something." I was tired of standing up for myself. *What difference will one more drug make?* I wondered. *I just want to get well. Please, God, don't make me live like this any longer.*

Chapter 13: The Treatment-Resistant Patient

Mom's experience with severe dental pain and depression launched my journey with understanding the mind-body connection. Though fully connecting that knowledge has taken time, I was beginning to put all of the pieces together with my experience of a chronic migraine. But no matter what I said, no doctor took me seriously enough to uncover the source of the pain. Or more likely, they simply lacked the tools to decipher the messages themselves. Some of them may have thought I had a psychosomatic illness. The bottom line is this: they lacked a model for understanding how the psyche communicates pain.

For example, when Mom's dentists heard her complaints of tooth and jaw pain, they investigated her teeth. They took x-rays, performed tests, proposed dental treatments, and prescribed pain meds. But their model was that if the pain was in the teeth and jaw, the problem had to be dental. I remember Dad saying that no one could figure out what was wrong with her teeth, because the x-rays and other tests failed to yield any concrete diagnostic information—the logical reason for a dentist to throw up his hands and suggest pulling all of her teeth.

According to a letter that Dad wrote to Mom's doctor before she was admitted to the hospital, she was taking Percodan (aspirin and oxycodone), Miltown (tranquilizer), NaButisol, and Pentobarbital (barbiturates). Additionally, Dad notes that one dentist who saw Mom refused to give her any medication because he thought she was overmedicated. No wonder Mom's psychiatrist insisted on detoxing her once she was admitted to the hospital. Mixing the drugs that Mom was taking can be dangerous and cause serious interactions, such as respiratory distress and central nervous system depression, especially when combined with alcohol.[32] Both *The Pill Book* and the website Drugs.com classify the drug interaction potential for these drugs as major and conclude that "the risk of interaction outweighs the benefit."

Mysterious pain is easily relegated to the margin when doctors use a dismissive term like "psychosomatic illness." Doctors can nod their collective heads at the patients, give them an antidepressant and an anti-anxiety drug, and tell them to come back in six months. Our Western medical model functions as if there is an impenetrable wall between the brain and the rest of the body—a person has either a mental illness or a physical illness. But in reality, we are one complex, interconnected system that operates with the goal of steering us toward wholeness.

Michael Greenwood and Peter Nunn, doctors specializing in the treatment of chronic pain, believe "all diseases have a physical, mental, emotional, spiritual, and environmental aspect...to begin to see the connection between mind and body is to begin to see the connection between all aspects of ourselves." Pain is often the mechanism that warns people that there is a problem—unrecognized distress with a life situation, the beginnings of a serious illness, a muscle or bone that is compromised in some way. All of these pains indicate the body's communication attempts. Sadly, not enough doctors look at pain with this understanding.[33]

And certainly not any of the doctors who were trying to help me. It seems to me that both Mom's doctors and, some twenty years later, my doctors, were all operating within the same paradigm: If one or two prescriptions don't work, then add a few more drugs. And many times, the doctors didn't discontinue any of the medications. Now doctors have a term for people like Mom and me, people for whom the drugs just don't work. They refer to us as *treatment resistant*—a term which sounds like blaming the patient for not getting well. Instead, why aren't they asking *If the treatment isn't working, could our approach be wrong?*

Some doctors *are* asking this question. In the past several years, clinicians have discovered that people taking antidepressants may improve initially, but then, after a time, they find their depression has worsened or even become chronic and irreversible (tardive dysphoria).[34] The idea of being stuck in a state of permanent despair is horrific to contemplate. Sadly, while this information is in the scientific literature, I have yet to see it covered in the mainstream media publications that most people read.

Chapter 14: A Therapeutic Environment

One May night in 1997, the night I'd returned from my second hospitalization that month to treat the migraine, the urge to kill myself competed for attention with the pledge I'd made to Dr. Sherman just a few weeks back: *I promise to check myself into the hospital if I ever decide to commit suicide.*

As I got dressed in the dark, walk-in closet, my heart raced. I pulled on a clean tee shirt and slipped on a pair of jeans, then grabbed a pair of sandals and tip-toed out of the bedroom. I didn't kiss Randy good-bye. Just minutes before, I'd been lying in bed with him after some perfunctory, "finally-home-from-the-hospital sex."

When we finished, he turned his back to me and said, "I guess our lives will always be like this."

"What do you mean?" I said, crossing my arms over my chest.

"You'll always be sick—in and out of the hospital—you're never going to get well."

A few minutes later, Randy was snoring away, while I lay on my back. Hot tears welled up in my eyes and rolled down my cheeks. No welcome home, no hugs of encouragement or whispers of how we were in this fight together. Just doom and gloom from the man I was spending my life with. In that moment, I saw no way out. For nearly the whole time I'd struggled with the migraine and depression, as one treatment morphed into another, interrupted by brief sparks of hope, I held firm to the belief that I'd get well, clinging to every possible hope. But not Randy. His prediction echoed in my ears: "You're just like your mother. You're always going to be sick."

Most of the time I fought back, ignoring him and using all of my mental, physical, and emotional tools to forge a path forward. But not now. Now escape seemed the only answer, and suicide my only route. But I didn't want to desert my kids.

I went upstairs, past the guest room where my in-laws were sleeping—they were visiting from Florida for a few days. I stood by Connor's bed and watched him as he slept on his side. Moonlight flooded his face. I kissed him on the forehead and walked out. I moved quietly to Eileen's room and did the same. She always made funny noises in her sleep and tonight was no different. As I kissed her cheek, I knew that I didn't want this kiss to be the last, but I was exhausted and out of hope. Going to the hospital seemed like the only option to save my life.

Imagine how humiliated you'd be if you went to the emergency room and the person at the admission desk was your former neighbor. Yes, that's who checked me in that night. I shared my darkest secret with the woman who hadn't spoken to me for years after her dog had bitten Eileen's lip. But tonight, she wore her game face and was actually pretty nice as she took down all of my medical information. Could things get any worse? Or more humiliating? No, I told myself. This is the hardest part. Until I met the social worker waiting for me in the cubicle.

"Ann, from what you're telling me, I think it would be a good idea to check you into the psych ward for a few days. That way, you can get some distance from the problems at home, maybe get some new meds, and begin to build yourself up again."

"New meds?" I was incredulous. "They kick in after four to six weeks, if they work at all."

A nurse stood next to her and nodded. "We're going to call Dr. Sherman for you. Would you like to speak to him?"

"Sure, but I don't want to stay tonight. I promise not to do anything to myself. I just need some help."

The nurse and the social worker looked at each other, raising their eyebrows.

Words tumbled out of my mouth. "I can't go into the hospital now. I just got home from another hospital for my headache treatments—it was the second time this month. My in-laws are staying with us, and this weekend my siblings and I are throwing a big party for our parents' sixtieth wedding anniversary. I can't stay here."

The nurse handed me the phone and I spoke to Dr. Sherman. "Hey," I said, "I just need some help. I promise not to hurt myself, but I can't stay here."

"Why not? Maybe you need to be in the hospital," he said.

I told him about the in-laws, the family party, the two recent hospitalizations. "I can't leave again. There's too much for me to take care of."

"Sounds like the perfect time to get away."

I smiled and swung my feet back and forth. "Look, I kept my promise to come to the hospital if I ever wanted to kill myself. Now I'm telling you that I won't. Please, I've got to go home." The time was creeping toward 1:00 a.m. I'd left the house around eleven o'clock, so probably no one even knew I was gone. "Look, I'll call you tomorrow. I'll check in every day until I can see you. Just tell them to let me go."

The nurse and social worker were waiting on the other side of the room, arms folded over their chests, looking down at the floor as if that gave me any privacy. I handed the phone to them. "He wants to talk to you."

The social worker left and spoke in hushed tones to Dr. Sherman and returned with some papers. "The doctor and I have agreed that if you'll sign this no-harm agreement, we'll release you, but you need to call him in the morning."

As I signed the agreement, I knew that I didn't really want to commit suicide—I wanted to escape the pain of dealing with Randy's pessimism. At the time, I don't think that I could allow myself to feel how unhappy I was and how impossible the whole marriage had become. In retrospect, I know that all of the drugs I was taking deadened my feelings, including the intense rage I felt toward Randy. There's even a name for the anesthetized feelings—psychic numbing. But back then, I thought my numbed-out state was a result of the prolonged depression. And as I drove home that night, I thought *I had a close call, but I'll be all right. I just need to get through the weekend.*

Despite being up for several hours in the middle of the night, I woke up about 6:30 the next morning to make coffee and breakfast for everyone. An empty refrigerator signaled to me that even though I'd been away all week, Randy hadn't gone to the store. He'd ordered take-out, buying time until I came home.

I threw on the clothes from the night before, grabbed my purse, and headed out to the store. As I raced through the aisles picking up strawberries, eggs, bacon, bread, and coffee, I felt really strange. *I feel the blood rushing in my veins.* Once I began driving, my heart raced and pounded. I had to keep moving, like I was supercharged with energy. Thoughts whirled in my brain like food in a blender. *Oh, God, maybe this is mania.*

I gripped the steering wheel and slowed down to the exact speed limit. I forced myself to think through the feelings. *I've been on Prednisone for weeks now, and twice with an IV. Could it be the drug or is it really mania?*[35] I knew two things: I had to call Dr. Sherman, and I had to tell Randy. I felt out-of-control.

"Where have you been?" my mother-in-law shouted at me as I walked in the kitchen door, arms loaded with groceries. "We've all been sitting around waiting for you so we can go to the strawberry festival." Martha had never yelled at me before. Randy, his father, Connor, and Eileen all stood next to her, looking down at the floor.

"I had to get groceries. There was nothing for breakfast, and I wanted to..." But Martha cut me off in mid-sentence.

"You're so inconsiderate. We all want to leave. Are you ready?"

My calm words were more and more of an effort as I felt my pulses screaming in my ears. *Oh, God, what's happening?*

"Sure, let me unload the groceries and talk to Randy first."

Martha stood beside me and started taking things out of bags and putting them away. "Go," was all she said.

I grabbed Randy by the arm and race-walked him down the hall to our bedroom, closing the door and taking him to the farthest corner of the room. "Look, there's no easy way to tell you this." He seemed to sense that something was very wrong.

"I'm out of control inside." I described the blood racing, the heart pounding. "I can literally feel the blood racing." He hugged me. "I need to call Dr. Sherman. I think I'm manic."

Then the impossible happened—Randy hugged me again. "Call him. I just want you to be OK. I'll deal with my parents and your family. You just need to get well." Randy squeezed my arm. "It'll be all right." And he walked out to face his parents and the kids.

I don't know what Randy told them, but Dr. Sherman and I agreed that he'd admit me to the hospital for observation, and that I was entering voluntarily. He didn't seem open to my idea about a reaction to Prednisone, but I was so upset, I let it go. I didn't even have time to think about the drastic move I was making. I was too terrified about what has happening inside of me.

But things in the kitchen were not pretty. Martha had put

away all of the groceries and was sipping on some coffee. Bob, her husband, sat next to her and squeezed my hand as I walked past him. Martha's tight jaw and twisted mouth signaled that Randy had delivered the news. Connor and Eileen had disappeared into their bedrooms like rabbits seeking safety from an impending thunderstorm.

"I'm sorry, but I need to go to the hospital again. I feel...," but before I could get the words out, Martha pounced.

"You are not sick. You just need to stay here and take care of your family."

I stood behind the island and faced Martha and Bob. "I don't know what Randy told you, but I feel out of control on the inside. I've never felt like this, and I'm scared," my words rushed out and the blood whooshed in my veins.

Martha fired another round: "You sure are messed up."

"Right back at you," tumbled out of my mouth. The first time I'd ever been remotely rude to my mother-in-law in all of my years of marriage.

Randy stood next to me and put his arm on my shoulder. "Come on, Ann, we need to go," He was kind to me in that moment, despite his mother's clear rage.

"YOU ARE NOT SICK!" Martha screamed as we walked out the door.

I was grateful to Randy for taking my side that day. As we drove to the hospital, we sat in silence. I never thought I'd find myself in this situation—ready to check into a psych hospital, but here I was. Dr. Sherman had told me that since he didn't have privileges at my local hospital, he'd find me another doctor to do the admission. "I know someone good who works there. You'll be fine," he'd promised. Another doctor, another opinion—I had no choice but to acquiesce.

A nurse showed Randy and me around the ward and then

led us to my room and introduced me to my roommate. "I'll keep your blow-dryer in the office, and if you need it in the morning, just ask," the nurse told me.

There was a curtain I could pull around my bed and a closet on the other side of the room. No privacy—security was the only concern as far as I could see. Randy pulled the curtains closed and we hugged and exchanged a brief kiss. "You'll be all right," he whispered. I held him tightly and squeezed back my tears.

"Thank you for being so supportive of me with your mother," I whispered to him. "It means a lot."

Randy squeezed my hand and kissed me before he turned to leave.

I awoke very early the next morning, showered, dressed, and tried to eat something at breakfast. I still felt racing in my body and my thoughts jumbled like clothes in the dryer. Sitting around a small table with several other patients, I marveled at the ease with which we talked to one another. I think what bonded us was the severity of our situation, and the fact that we'd all endured some kind of trauma that had landed us in a locked psych ward.

The routine of the inpatient unit was nearly identical to the routine in the outpatient unit—breakfast at 8:00, Goals Group at 9:00, and then expressive therapy at 10:00. Again, I fit right in with the arrangement of the days, thanks to my twelve years of Catholic school regimentation and the ability to say yes and smile no matter how I really felt. I wondered what my goal might be—besides getting out of the hospital. One patient gave her goal as maintaining for the day, so I realized that my goal could be simple. I don't remember what I said the first day, but one day when I was still feeling manic and very playful, I joked with a few men at breakfast that my goal for the day was to get laid. But the only man I was attracted to had left that afternoon, so I never acted on my manic impulses. Knowing me, I doubt that I would have, but it was fun to be so free.

Just like what you see in the movies, patients stood in a

medication line several times a day. The nurses barricaded themselves behind a glass wall where they handed out the white cups of pills and monitored us patients to be sure we swallowed them. The décor was shabby-clinical, with pale green walls and scattered prints of non-descript artwork, the kind you might see in a hotel. The dayroom looked like a family room in a house with lots of kids—boxes of board games scattered on shelves, worn, upholstered furniture, and several straight-backed chairs, the kind you see in waiting rooms and school offices. The unit's atmosphere was as cold as the staff, who seemed more like easily spooked horses than the nurturing helpers that I'd always thought psych nurses would be.

I wondered why the nurses needed to be behind glass for so much of the day. Who was being protected from whom? Were we as patients dangerous? I guess at times some people were, but in the five days that I was hospitalized, I never saw anyone act out. In fact, I think we were all pretty well sedated, so we went along with the inane bullshit of the routine. Bullshit that included cameras trained on us at meals, smoke breaks on a small porch, dictatorial nurses threatening to take away our meds or to put one of us in the quiet room. I remembered what Dr. Sherman had told me about some of his patients being restrained—strapped and shackled to their beds—so I knew that violence from the nurses was a very real possibility. I harbored no desire to test the limits. I also remembered that Randy had told me he'd built the "quiet room" in this hospital, and I was not about to do or say anything that might land me in a room with a mat on the floor and padded walls.

In order to be hospitalized as an inpatient, you needed to be in pretty dire straits, as most of the other patients revealed. I met a woman consumed with suicidal feelings, probably as a result of severe depression after giving up drinking. Another woman had no family in the state and lived in a windowless basement apartment. She wore long-sleeve blouses all the time to hide her cutting. And one of the men had been gang-raped as a teen. Instead of support and understanding for his chronic anxiety and depression, his father mocked his pain.

Looking back on this experience, I'm struck by the lack of

processing that the doctors and nurses offered us. In general, they were more focused on "stabilizing" us on meds and less focused on how to help us better cope with our traumas. Why didn't the hospital offer patients assistance in exploring our complex situations? Why weren't we encouraged to craft new strategies for our return home?

Instead of tailoring sessions for small groups or even individuals, our group therapy consisted of bland, generic offerings related to building better coping mechanisms. Why weren't we working on some role-playing to assist us with problem situations when we got home? Why didn't the staff teach us some cognitive-based therapy? The deeper forms of support took place as we patients talked and shared our own stories, outside of group. And all of us needed more than a few adjustments with our medications, which is pretty much all the hospital had to offer.

Oddly enough, no matter how many times doctors and nurses talked with me about my recent history and what was going on in my life, no one made the connection between taking Prednisone for three weeks and my feelings of mania. Now I know that I wasn't experiencing mania as part of a bipolar episode. I was experiencing the effects of taking Prednisone, a powerful steroid, for over three weeks, including one week of an IV infusion in the hospital. The warnings about mania are clearly written on the pill packaging. Adverse reactions to report to your doctor include agitation, euphoria, headache, and fast, pounding, or irregular heartbeat, among others.

But my records contained the diagnosis—thanks to "the Hopkins doctor"—that I experienced mild, atypical, hypomania along with depression. Dr. Sherman referred to my diagnosis as Bipolar II, the less extreme form of bipolar disorder. So, everyone treated me as if I had bipolar disorder, and I went along with it, because to express doubt or to question a doctor got you labelled as a difficult patient.

I wonder what might have happened if, instead of hospitalizing me, someone had spoken to me about the effects of Prednisone and the possibility of manic symptoms. Would there have been another treatment? Hospitalization is certainly an expensive and drastic way to deal with a medication response, but maybe that's more common that I know.

In comparison to the other patients, I remember feeling like my situation was the best of anyone's—headache and all. Even though I was a patient in a psych ward, I knew that I could go home to kids who loved me and friends who supported me. I had a comfortable life and a beautiful home. Randy was another matter—but at the time, I don't think I saw our relationship as the biggest hurdle in my life. I was so used to struggling with him and compromising on problems and even lying to him so that he'd get off my back, that I couldn't see that the constant stress of trying to please him and avoid his criticism was deeply harmful. After twenty-two years of marriage and therapy on and off for about seventeen years, I had resigned myself to coping as best I could. And while Martha's awful words still rang in my head, I pushed them aside and hoped that all we'd shared in the years before would help us to heal this recent rift.

My biggest insight about being in a psych hospital still rings true to me today, even though I wrote these words over twenty years ago:

> *The irony of mental illness is striking and forceful: the ones who perpetrate the abuse or harm a person in their formative years often get off without any retribution. Yet the abused are left with a ravished psyche and some form of depression or passionate-desperation [bipolar disorder] that descends upon them at very stressful times in their lives. The victims bear the stigma of illness, not the sick ones who inflicted harm on us. Harm so severe [that in some cases] our psyches are forever scarred, and we are left with illnesses that are more terrifying than anything that Steven King could imagine or design. The injured ones become the strong simply because we survived the first attacks and are asked to defend against more for the rest of our lives. I saw courage on a grand scale in that hospital, courage to match any ever seen on a field of battle. We fought the ultimate battles against darkness, rage, and fear. We, the mentally ill ones, are the true heroes.*

Chapter 15: Slow-walking to the Inevitable

Sometime late in 1997, a few months after my sojourn in the psych ward, the depression lifted for more than a few days. By that time, along with the numerous combinations of meds I'd consumed, I'd endured seven ECT treatments of four shocks each, equivalent to twenty-eight individual treatments. I never could have made myself go through the whole procedure that many times, so I was grateful that Dr. Sherman used the four-shock method. Happily, a few days turned into a few weeks, and when I'd felt really good every day for about a month, I sensed that my long, dark night was finally over.

But when people ask me how I got well, I tell them that I honestly don't know. I think my recovery was largely driven by an iron will and unshakeable belief in myself, an intuitive knowledge that my journey was about something deep and profound in my psyche, plus a strong commitment to show Randy—and myself—that I would never be like my mother. And when Dr. Sherman insisted that I stay on all of my psych meds for an indeterminate period of time, I agreed, grateful to finally be well and determined to do whatever it took to stay in the light.

But the battle to regain my soul wasn't over; it had simply shifted to a new frontier: my marriage. And I can pinpoint the event that marked the turn.

About two years earlier, midway into the four years of depression, Randy and I argued heatedly about whether or not I was working hard enough to regain my health. Early one morning, I was dressed in my exercise gear, ready to go for a walk, and Randy came down from his office to find something. I remember light pouring in through the window overlooking the woods behind our house. I remember the soft green of the leaves. And I remember our conversation.

"Good thing you're going for a walk. Maybe it'll make you feel better, though I doubt it," Randy said as he rummaged in his dresser.

"Randy, I know I'm going to get well. It's just taking longer than we hoped."

I risked sharing an insight that I'd had that morning when I prayed and drew an angel card, a source of inspiration for my day. "Today I drew a card with an angel standing on top of a mountain holding a little white flag. My word for today is *surrender*..." Before I could explain, Randy cut me off.

"Surrender? Oh, great, now you're giving up." He slammed the drawer and turned to face me. "Well, I gave up a long time ago. You're hopeless, and now you won't even fight anymore." He walked toward the door to leave.

"Randy, wait, you don't understand," I begged. "To me, *surrender* means acceptance of what *is*—not fighting reality, but flowing with it until things change."

He pounded his fist on the door and then turned and faced me. "You're just like your mother. You're going to be depressed forever. I never know what I'm coming home to. Will you be in bed? Will you feel good? Maybe tell me the meds are working? Or will you have that hideous scarf wrapped around your head with the blue ice pack?"

His words hit me—a barrage of bullets. Hot tears leaked from my eyes. "Randy, listen to me..."

He cut me off. "Well, I've heard it all before. Each new pill—you think it's going to work. Now the doctors say you're bipolar. Why didn't you ever hear that before?"

"Randy, I take care of everything in the house, do all the cooking, watch out for the kids, run my sewing business…" My voice trailed off. How many times had we had this conversation? How else could I show that I was keeping things together? "I'm not like my mother. She couldn't even…"

"Just stop!" he yelled. "It's been years of this mess screwing with our lives. My drinking problem was one thing, but this depression? The migraine? Our kids will be scarred forever."

"Randy, please." I wiped my face. "I'm doing my best. Please believe me. I know I'll get well." I moved toward him, reaching for his shoulder.

His body stiffed and his cheeks flamed. "This wasn't in the contract when we got married. I never signed up for this."

I buckled inside as if I'd been punched. I stared at him.

Randy stood in the doorway, ready to leave. "Just go away, Ann. Maybe that's what you need. We could all manage without you." He walked a few steps down the hall, then turned back and looked at me. "Come back when you're normal."

Randy's boots thudded on the tile floor as he walked away. When I heard the click of the lock, I collapsed on the bed and sobbed for a long time until I felt sick and exhausted. Randy had been angry with me many times before, but it had been months since he'd hurled such hurtful words. I felt so drained that I couldn't imagine going for a walk. I decided to do what I always did when I was upset and needed to process—I wrote in my journal.

As my words appeared on the computer screen, I remembered some of the angry things that my father had said to Mom, although he'd never been as mean as Randy. I read his words over again. "I didn't sign up for this." "We can manage without you." "Come back when you're normal." And I don't know where this thought came from, but a voice inside me said, *That's not anger. That's abuse.*

The thought of someone verbally abusing me triggered something inside, and I knew what I needed to do. I marched up to Randy's office, not knowing what I would say, but determined to set a firm boundary. I wasn't going to let myself live as an abused woman—now that I could see what was going on.

My mind flooded with what I wanted to say to him. And one thing Randy had said was stuck as if on a repeating loop—"My drinking problem was one thing…" He'd simply tossed that phrase out as if he were talking about his bike. But I remembered all the nights I'd made dinner and he didn't call, coming home drunk at nine or ten o'clock and then falling asleep on the sofa. Or the parties we'd attended where he'd find a way to make me the brunt of his humor so that everyone laughed at me. And the car accident when he totaled our car—drunk on beer and high on pot—while I was pregnant. Or the day he was stoned and drinking beer and letting Connor use a table saw. We'd been over that territory, and even though he'd stopped drinking, he'd never addressed the underlying issues—he'd simply switched obsessions from drinking to tennis, to over-work, and now to biking. But I knew if I compared the damage his addiction issues had done to our marriage to my struggles with depression, we'd never address the issue staring us in the face.

When I walked into the office, Randy raised his eyebrows and looked up from his computer. "All those awful things you said to me—that's not anger, Randy. That's verbal abuse. And I won't allow it any more. You need to go get help, and you need to stop speaking to me that way. I'm not going to stay in a marriage where I'm being abused."

I felt my shoulders relax as I spoke to him. I don't know where my courage came from. While I'd been a crying heap a few hours ago, now I was standing up to my husband. "You need to go to therapy, Randy. I don't deserve the way you spoke to me."

He looked down at the floor and then locked eyes with me.

"Ann, I'm so sorry. I'm just so worried about you. I'm frustrated that you're still sick after all the doctors and medications. I promise I won't speak to you like that again. What can I do to make it up to you?"

"Go to therapy," I repeated. I thought that making that demand was all it would take. I set a boundary and told him to stop--the same way I'd told him many things before. But the weight of the word abuse made me realize that we were in a crisis situation. Randy was working with a therapist in a men's group that he attended once a week. He didn't say much about what went on, but he seemed to get a lot out of it, so I suggested he talk to his therapist. The verbal abuse was *his* problem. All I had to do was wait for him to straighten out. *Then* we'd be OK.

Of course, things got better for a while, just like they always did, and then they slipped back. Time and again, Randy would fire off more awful things at me, and I would set another boundary. We'd tried couples therapy many times, but he'd always set a limit for how many times he'd go with me. And even though Randy and I had periods of time where we got along well and even enjoyed time with each other, the longer we were married, the more rarely those times occurred.

I don't know what he and his therapist discussed, but it didn't seem like Randy was making much progress. Not only did he continue to disparage me, he criticized things that most people wouldn't even have a conversation about. Petty things—like the mops and brooms I used.

The first floor in our house was tiled, so I swept and mopped frequently, because we lived in the woods, and everyone tracked in dirt. I used a straw-bristle broom, just like my mother had used, just like I'd been using for all of the years that Randy and I were married. One day, he came down from his office to the house for lunch when I was sweeping the floors, and for some reason, he didn't like the broom.

"That's the wrong broom for this kind of floor, Ann. You need a soft-bristle broom to sweep tile floors."

I laughed. "I've been using this same kind of broom ever since we moved in here. You've never said it was a problem before."

"Well, now I am. You need to get the proper broom. You'll see a difference," he assured me.

I didn't rush out that day to get a new broom, but after he nagged me about it a few more times, I bought the kind he recommended. But it still wasn't right. I tried two or three more brooms, and we had similar conversations about the mop I used to wash the floor. Randy said that the kind I was using just pushed the dirt around the floor while another kind was too cumbersome; I needed one that was more compact and designed for tile. I still don't know what kind of mop is designed for tile.

Finally, after months of criticism about the mops and brooms, I'd had enough. "Randy, let's go to the hardware store together, and you can show me the right kind of mop and broom. Then we can be done with this discussion." I thought I'd devised the perfect solution.

"Ann, if you can't figure out the right kinds of mops and brooms to buy, then I don't know what to say. I don't have time to go shopping with you." We were at a complete stand-off, over mops and brooms. I decided to ignore his comments the next time and just keep offering my solution.

Looking back on our relationship, I can see a pattern in Randy's criticisms that I didn't recognize when we were married. We had the same kinds of arguments about travel, where he'd criticize my driving, often yelling at me until I cried, and then telling me if I couldn't drive right, the least I could do is read the map and navigate. Then he'd yell at me if I didn't read the map correctly and grab it out of my hands in disgust. After numerous trips where this problem occurred, I proposed a solution that I'd worked out with my therapist, Fran.

"Randy, let's sit down a couple of nights before we leave on vacation and go over the map. I'll highlight the route and write down the directions step-by-step. That way, I can be prepared, and we can avoid an argument."

His answer had a familiar ring to it. "I don't have time for that, Ann. If you can't read a map and help me out, I don't know what to say. Besides, I don't want to lock in a route, and then that's all you know. What if there's a detour? You need to work on your map-reading skills."

After years of this travel-scenario, I began to dread any kind of trip with Randy. I went to therapy several weeks before a trip and worked out coping plans and responses with my therapist. And while I laughed about it with my friends, I knew that it wasn't normal to dread going on vacation with your husband and to have to armor yourself against his biting remarks. In fact, I often planned trips alone to visit my brother and cousin in California or my friend in Utah. I frequently went away to a retreat center for five days at a time to give myself a break. The distance I felt from him only increased over the years, as did my resentment at the way he continued to belittle me.

And we continued to have conversations about his verbal abuse—which became more and more frequent. By the time my depression had lifted, I didn't love him anymore, but I knew I couldn't leave him because I continued to struggle with daily migraine pain. I remember one session with my therapist Pauline that clarified my dilemma. I shared some stories with her about the travel issues and the mop-and-broom debate, as well as a similar scenario where I'd contact Randy on his pager, his office phone, and his cell phone, but he'd never return my calls. Then when I'd ask him why he didn't get back to me he'd say, "Everyone else knows how to get ahold of me. What's the matter with you?"

After we both shook our heads in disbelief, Pauline asked me, "Can you see yourself with him when you're seventy-five?"

"Ha! I can't see myself with him when I'm fifty-five." And as soon as those words popped out of my mouth, I knew divorce loomed as a solution. But I wasn't ready to give up, and I couldn't work because of the pain. During our twenty-plus years of marriage, we'd always had a fractious relationship. Things would get better after I got rid of my migraine. That's what I told Pauline—and myself. I played that conversation with Pauline over and over in my head as I worked around the house. My stomach lurched every time Randy's boots thudded in the hall, or he barked my name as he walked in the door as if I'd done something wrong. Even the kids noticed and would sometimes imitate their father just to see me jump.

In retrospect, I think the two situations that stand out in my mind as creating an unbridgeable gap between Randy and me were his obsession with biking and the family trip we took to Ireland in 1999. Eileen had asked me a few years back what interests Randy and I shared when we fell in love. I paused for a moment and then said, "Camping and biking."

We both laughed, because by the time I'd gone camping with Connor as a toddler while pregnant with Eileen, and then camping while taking care of two children under five, I'd completely sworn it off. In fact, my stomach churned every time Randy told me about his dream for our retirement: "We'll buy a pop-up camper and then drive around the country together." *Great, my two most hated things—camping and driving with Randy.*

My instinctive dread didn't bode well for spending our golden years together. And as for biking, once the kids had come along, the only way I could bike was to use a child-seat, which made it really hard to peddle up hills. And after having two children, my hips had spread a bit and the bike seat was very uncomfortable.

I hadn't biked for over fifteen years when Randy announced he was taking up biking. "It's something that I can share with Connor."

Connor had joined the biking club at his high school and had placed in several races. At first, I thought it would be a great way for the two of them to spend father-son time together; instead, the biking turned into a fierce competition to see who could ride the fastest.

Connor's club did a lot of trail-riding in state parks, so there were always branches to ride over and ditches in the path to jump. Riders joked about doing an "endo," which means hitting a ditch or a branch and then being pitched headfirst over the handle bars. Dislocated shoulders were common among bikers, as were broken collarbones. Randy found a group of much younger men and began riding with them at least twice a week. In fact, he never missed a Saturday in the last five years of our marriage. And when we had an argument or found ourselves at an impasse, Randy would jump on his bike and ride away.

He loved biking so much that I nicknamed his bike "Sweetie," joking that she never said no and was always ready to accommodate his needs. I went so far as to suggest that he park "Sweetie" in our bedroom. On the holidays, Randy rode his bike every spare moment. "What time is your family coming over?" he'd ask before he left the house. He'd schedule his return home so that he had just enough time to shower and change before the guests arrived. The kids and I were left with all of the cleaning and meal preparation while Randy could act as the affable host and then complain about doing the dishes once all of the guests had left.

The longer Randy and I were married, the more we'd grown in different directions. He was never much of a reader, other than the magazines *Architectural Design* and *Popular Mechanics.* I can remember only one book that he read: *The 7 Habits of Highly Effective People*, while I read nonfiction books about the environment and politics, plus every novel and book about spirituality that I could find.

One night when we were lying in bed, Randy asked, "Have you seen my dirt rag?"

"No," I said. "Why the heck would you keep a dirt rag in the bedroom?"

"It's a biking magazine called *Dirt Rag*, not an actual rag. Don't you know that?"

We weren't even speaking the same language any more.

And then there was the family trip to Ireland that we took

in July of 1999. Randy had been to Ireland with his parents before we got married, but that was nearly twenty-five years ago. Connor and Eileen were in their late teens, which we figured was the ideal time to take them to Europe. I spent months planning the trip, checking out airfares, and finding cute B and Bs where we could stay. We landed in Shannon and then used buses and trains as we toured several towns on the coast and then on to the Ring of Kerry, which wove through Kilarney National Park. One place that the kids and I wanted to see was Blarney Castle, but since Randy had already been there with his parents, he didn't want to go. We had the same discussion repeatedly for a few days before we arrived in the town nearest to Blarney Castle.

"Ann, I've already been there. Why should I waste my time going again? Besides, I've been checking out some nice bike rides."

"Randy, I've never been there and neither have the kids. You can ride your bike any time. Please go with us."

"You can take a bus with the kids. I'm going for a bike ride," he announced.

Deserted once again, I was determined to make the day a memorable one for Connor and Eileen. I knocked on the door of their room and gave them the news. "Your dad's not coming to Blarney Castle with us, but we're going to have a wonderful day, so I'm sorry he'll miss out." It was tough not to put Randy down in front of the kids, but they probably read my disappointment.

They didn't say anything to me, but their blank faces told me how they felt. While we waited for the bus and chatted about our day, Randy walked toward us without a bike by his side.

"I decided to come after all," he announced. "It's not a good day for a bike ride—probably going to rain."

While I was happy that he'd joined us, I couldn't quiet the voice inside that was practically screaming, "This is a family vacation. We need to spend time as a family, not doing things separately. How can you be so selfish?"

Randy enjoyed the day and had the traditional Blarney Castle picture taken, lying down on a rock and bending back to kiss the Blarney Stone. I hid my feelings behind a practiced smile, but anger and disappointment seethed inside, because a seemingly simple thing like spending the day with your family in Ireland required so much negotiation, even begging, to finally arrive at a yes.

Many evenings, the kids and I were alone because Randy went off on a bike ride and didn't return until nearly 11:00 pm. I was usually in bed when he got back, and then he'd go off to dinner in a local pub. So, while I loved being in Ireland and spending time exploring with the kids, I felt increasingly disconnected from Randy. As he pulled away from spending time with us, I'd negotiate for more of his time, just like I did at home.

Now, when I think of that trip to Ireland, a heavy blanket of sadness wraps itself around me, because I'd begun to see that the gulf between Randy and me was nearly insurmountable.

I wanted more out of life, more out of my marriage. I resented Randy and felt distant from him, tired of defending myself from his constant attacks on my health and the medications I took. We went through the motions of marriage, but my heart wasn't in it. Because I was still gripped with migraine pain and taking numerous drugs, I felt trapped; the path to a new life was shrouded in a mist as thick and impenetrable as the white fog rising from the Irish Sea. It would take a miracle, or maybe an angel, for me to find my way.

Chapter 16: From Pollyanna to Polypharmacy

"Lady, are you all right?" I woke up suddenly. A man in a dark leather jacket pounded on my driver's side window.

A pungent smell filled the car. I felt the airbag pushing me against my seat, wedging me in place. *Must wake up.* The man pounded on the window again. I rolled it down and looked at him through heavy-lidded eyes.

"I'm so drugged."

"Lady, don't ever say that again."

The cold air rushing into the car jolted me awake. What had happened? I saw a black van stopped inches away from the front of my car. Traffic crawled and then crept past us. I was pinned behind the airbag, but, somehow, I managed to free myself and get out of the car. We stood in the middle of Route 40, the main thoroughfare through Baltimore, surveying the damage. The man's van didn't have a scratch on it, but the front of my little Toyota was pretty banged up.

Before I could ask him any questions, he ordered me back into my car. "Park in one of those empty spaces," he directed, motioning to the lot next to our crash site. He hopped into his van and led me to a parking spot.

I think the man in the dark jacket asked me if I was all right, but I was dazed, or more likely, in a stupor. I expected him to be angry, but, instead, he patiently waited in the cold with me. I can't remember if I had a cell phone, but I must have. Did I give it to the man and ask him to call my father? Maybe.

In a few minutes my dad arrived, and I think he talked to the man in the dark jacket. Dad hugged me and wanted to know if I was OK. *At least he wasn't angry with me.*

What just happened? No one had been hurt, but my car was banged up. *Randy's going to kill me*, reverberated in my mind when I imagined the inevitable confession to my husband. My neck began to hurt, but I don't think I cried.

"I have to give that man my insurance information," I told Dad, and fumbled in the glove compartment, looking for the documents. But when I found them and got out of the car, the man in the dark jacket was gone. He never asked for my name or phone number. To this day, I swear he was an angel.

"Come on home, Ann. We'll talk there and get you warmed up," Dad said.

Still dazed, I wondered *Am I in shock?* I remember going to my parents' house and having tea with them. Their calm demeanors and kind words masked any worry they may have felt.

As I sat in the familiar yellow kitchen of my childhood home, both hands cupped around the steaming tea mug, I began to piece together the events of that afternoon. My mind raced as my parents' voices faded into the background. I knew that people walked in between cars all the time on Route 40, especially when traffic was stopped. What if a pedestrian had been between the van and my car? At the very least, I could have hurt someone badly. Was I going fast or had I slowed down? There must have been some momentum for the airbag to explode like that. Maybe I fell asleep before I put on the brakes? *Oh, God, I could have killed someone.* And like every other drunk or drug addict, I would walk away without an injury. And someone else would pay for my carelessness.

This accident was my second in the past few months. The other one had been even worse—I had repeatedly fallen asleep on Route 70 heading west to Frederick—again in the afternoon—and swerved across the highway five times. I finally lost control of the car and then crashed into a guardrail. A woman and her daughter pulled over. *Oh, God, did I hurt someone?* They walked toward me. Standing next to my Toyota, I wrapped my arms in front of my body and shivered. *What should I say to them?*

Instead of an angry snarl, the woman's voice was soft, her face etched with concern. "Can you make it home?" she asked. My front bumper dangled like a needle on a thread. "We saw you zig-zag across the highway. Are you all right?"

"Did I hit your car? I asked, very confused as to why they had stopped. She assured me that the only damage was to my vehicle, but that she was alarmed by my erratic driving.

"I'm OK," I lied. But my icy, shaking hands told another story. What the hell had happened to me? I'd never lost control of my car before. And, I'd never been on so many drugs before.

When the second car accident happened in January of 2000, I was driving to my parents' house for my weekly visit after volunteering in a depression support program at Johns Hopkins Hospital. I worked in their office on Mondays answering the phone and assisting people from all over the country who struggled with serious emotional distress. I helped them find doctors, therapists, and support groups. I empathized with the callers and had good listening skills, so they seemed to enjoy talking to me. But most of all, I felt useful. And despite my own struggles with depression, I could finally say that I was well. No symptoms for the past three years, and my psychiatrist kept me loaded up with Wellbutrin, Elavil, Valium, and Topamax as a precaution against another episode. I felt pretty good most days—except for my migraine.

Though I took numerous drugs to control it, the pain only subsided briefly when my dentist first prescribed Valium. Several subsequent doctors also prescribed Valium, but nothing alleviated the agony for more than a few hours. The doctors were more concerned about treating my depression and shrugged at me when I complained about the constant migraine.

Despite five hospitalizations that lasted about a week each and included IV Prednisone along with ever-increasing doses of pain drugs, I still had a constant migraine. At the time of my second accident, my headache remedies included daily doses of Methadone and DHE-45 injections, along with Imitrex nasal spray. Due to some serious bruising, my thighs couldn't take the needles, so I administered the injections to my hips. Blood vessels had ruptured, resulting in large, purple and blue blotches that my underwear barely covered. For the days when all I could do was lie in bed with a big, blue ice-pack tied to my head, I had injectable Demerol.

And taking Methadone—that was a move of pure desperation. All of my meds were by prescription; I didn't ever feel high or happy taking them. My nurse practitioner had previously prescribed MS-Contin (morphine) and then OxyContin, a new opioid that was supposed to be highly effective and non-addictive. Neither of them stopped the anguish. In fact, I thought that they stopped working because the pain increased. I was terribly ashamed about taking Methadone, a medication that I thought belonged in the hands of a *drug addict*. In my mind, that was someone who used drugs, illegally, and for pleasure. So, by my definition, I was no drug addict.

But I felt badly shaken by this second car accident. Two serious car crashes in less than six months. I thought about how my dad had taken away my mother's license when she'd had two or three accidents in a row—also in the afternoon, and usually after drinking a beer at lunchtime along with all of her daily psych meds. *I've hit rock bottom*, I realized. Western medicine had failed me.

"Betty, I need the phone number for that energy healer you talked about a few months ago," I confessed to my friend about the two accidents and hoped she still had the contact information.

Betty gave me the number and said, "Ann, working with Kayla provided me with the deepest healing I've ever had. I know she can help you." After I hung up, I remember feeling like I was about to do something bold—like sky-diving on a rainy night. *Nothing else is working*, I told myself as I dialed Kayla's number. When she answered, I poured out my story and begged for her help.

"I can almost guarantee you that I'll help you get rid of your headache," Kayla said, "but I can't guarantee what else might happen. Are you ready?"

"Yes."

I don't remember asking how much it cost to work with her, where I had to go to see her, or how long it would take to rid me of the pain. None of that mattered. We set up an appointment for later in the week. Kayla asked me a series of questions about my health and my personal situation. She asked me about my marriage, and I must have indicated that I was more and more unhappy—even questioning if I wanted to stay. Kayla said, "Don't you want to work on your relationship?"

I didn't hesitate. "No," I told her. "I've been working on my marriage for twenty years. I want to work on me."

Working with Kayla required my time, a good bit of money, and most of all, my faith in the unseen. Every treatment consisted of talking with her on the phone about how I was feeling, the names and doses of my meds, then hanging up and relaxing in my bed for about an hour while Kayla performed what she called *distance energy healing*. Kayla lived in a northern Baltimore County neighborhood, about forty-five miles from my home.

"I clear your chakras," she explained, "and sometimes I get messages from higher beings, or I see strange images inside your body." I didn't know what the heck *chakras* were, but I started reading about them so that I could understand her explanations when we spoke on the phone after each healing.

After I accumulated a rudimentary understanding of the chakras, Kayla's work made much more sense in relation to the kinds of physical and emotional issues that had dogged me for much of my life. Chakras, I learned, are energy centers throughout the body that can be shut down by stress and emotional or physical problems and can be recharged by cosmic energy, like healing touch. For example, Kayla frequently saw images and did a lot of clearing in my third chakra, also known as the throat chakra. This chakra is related to speaking your truth and expressing anger and other emotions in a constructive manner—a persistent problem for me, especially with Randy. I can remember times when I was so filled with rage that I wanted to explode, yet no matter what I said to him or how often we went to therapy, the dynamic between us stayed the same—he accused me of being too sensitive or too depressed or too serious. The problems, in his mind, were always my fault.

So, I found a physical release for my pent-up fury and frustration. Once a week or so I'd go out into the woods behind our house, pick up a heavy, dead branch, and whack the hell out of some poor oak tree while I cursed and shouted Randy's name. Then I'd apologize to the tree and come back into the house so I could journal away the rest of the pain.

But after Kayla and I had worked together for a month or so, she remarked after a healing, "Today I pulled out yards of cotton stuffing from the third chakra and then filled it with blue light, the color for that chakra. Does that image mean anything to you?" We both laughed when I told her about my "anger management" strategy.

"The cotton stuffing is all of the things I'm afraid to say to Randy. It makes perfect sense that my throat would be filled with some kind of blockage."

The other chakra from which she frequently saw images and received messages during a healing was the solar plexus—located right above the abdomen. I learned that when it's out of balance, you're sensitive to rejection and may suffer from eating disorders. I could say a loud Amen to those issues—I'd always been called "too sensitive," especially by Randy, and had suffered from eating disorders for many years during my late teens and early twenties.

With Kayla's help over several sessions, I began to feel more balanced and had a greater sense of my personal power. She also urged me to protect my solar plexus region whenever I was near anyone who threatened me in some way. "Hold a notebook or place a folder in front of the chakra. Make sure you sit sideways so you're not in a direct line with all of the person's negative energy." It didn't take me long to figure out that I needed to do that when Randy and I talked about anything contentious or when he said mean things to me. And as the migraine pain receded, I found it easier to set boundaries. And I was less willing to put up with his attempts to control me.

"I'm going to make you some flower essences to help keep your vibration strong," Kayla told me after the first few sessions. "Put a few drops of each in your water and then sip the mixture all day," she directed.

"What are flower essences and how can they help me?" I asked. I was still taking Methadone for the pain, for God's sake, so what the heck could these essence things do for me? But something compelled me to take Kayla's advice—I was all in and ready to risk something completely foreign in the hopes that I could finally get rid of the migraine. Skepticism was quickly shoved aside by an insistent voice inside saying, *Nothing else is working. At least these things won't make you sleepy.*

Kayla started me on two well-known blends: Self Heal and Five Flower. She explained, "Doctor Bach was a British physician disillusioned with Western medicine. He wanted to find natural remedies to help people improve their health and discovered that the essences of various flowers have healing properties—both physically and emotionally. Have you ever heard of Bach's Rescue Remedy? Health food stores often sell it—it's wonderful for anxiety."

"How will they help me?"

"Self Heal can support all of the work that we're doing to help you marshal your inner resources. It works to support a healthy mind-body connection. And Five Flower is an all-around formula that promotes physical and emotional healing in addition to relieving stress and tension."

"Whatever you say, Kayla. I want to get off of all of these dangerous meds. They're not helping the pain, and the side effects are awful." Each time Kayla talked about the mind-body connection, a little more insight wedged itself into my consciousness. I began to wonder if the headache really was my psyche's way of signaling deep distress. Distress that I couldn't admit.

As we continued to work together, Kayla concocted custom mixes of flower essences for me to take, along with Five Flower and Self Heal. She'd always give me a brief explanation of what the essences were supposed to do, and I took them religiously, mixing the tinctures in with the water I sipped all day. After about a month of working together, I still had pain, but it wasn't as grinding as it had been. I was getting better, finally. And then we embarked on tapering off of the migraine drugs one by one.

My memory of this time is fragmented: Methadone, Valium, Wellbutrin—all of them can cloud your mind. I don't know how Kayla learned about drug tapering, but I trusted her more than my doctors. Even so, I'm sure I consulted with my nurse practitioner about tapering, because I knew I had to keep her in the loop. But unlike so many of the doctors I'd worked with, Kayla actually listened to me, and she was able to help me make sense of all the internal changes I was experiencing. Because I was getting results, I willingly followed her suggestions.

As I reduced one drug—probably the Methadone—I remember experiencing several nights of grueling insomnia, tossing, turning, and finally sitting upright in a chair all night, waiting for the sun. But the pain was lessening. And my psychiatrist was willing to give me a small supply of Ambien to get through the crisis. Stopping Ambien had its own problems, but by then I had discovered melatonin, so after a few rough nights and groggy days, I began to sleep well again.

I remember using the blue ice-packs less and less as the pain faded and seemed to take up an increasingly smaller area of my scalp. I continued to see my nurse practitioner once a month to apprise her of my progress. She seemed supportive but more than a little skeptical when I told her about the flower essences. She'd smile and wish me well, and while I'll never know her true thoughts, it was hard to argue with my success. After seven years of grueling pain, I began to believe that I could wake up one morning without a migraine.

By May of 2000, four months after my auto accident, Kayla and I accomplished the goal I had set for myself—to heal my migraine and get off of all the pain medications. When I saw my headache nurse for my final visit, she was amazed that I was not only pain-free, but that I had also been able to withdraw from all of the drugs fairly easily. I continued taking the maintenance depression medications, even though three years had passed since my last bout with darkness.

I felt confident and strong, surer of myself and more secure in my ability to set boundaries and get what I needed. I was more able to stand up to my psychiatrist and challenge him when things weren't working. More able to stand up to Randy and refuse to accept any abusive behavior or disparaging remarks. After years of struggle and pain, I finally had the tools I needed to rebalance and move on. But I never thought that moving on would have such a literal meaning until a sunny afternoon in the middle of May. Just two weeks before we were to leave on our twenty-fifth anniversary trip.

Chapter 17: Trust Your Inner Voice

I was filled with mixed feelings about our marriage, but even so, we'd made plans a few months back to visit Eleuthera, an island in the Bahamas.

Randy and I were moving winter clothes up to the storage room and bringing down summer clothes, a ritual requiring a lot of lifting and many trips up and down the stairs. After I'd seen him empty-handed a few times, I said, "Randy, could you please be sure to carry clothes on each end of the trip? We'll get done a lot faster."

He kicked a box of clothes across the room and pounded his fist on the wall. Then he yelled at me and stormed out of the house, slamming the front door. *Where did that come from?* I wondered, as I stood in the bedroom.

Even though Randy had done things like that many times before, on that day, I felt different. Realizing it was useless to confront him, I completed the clothing transfer on my own, which took me about an hour. When I finished, I sat in a rocking chair in the upstairs family room. The house was quiet. Both kids were out with their friends, and Randy was still up in his office or on a bike ride. I'd only been sitting up there alone for a while when I heard him come through the front door and bound up the stairs.

He knelt down in front of me and said, "I'm so sorry for the way I acted. I was way off base. I'm going to make you a nice dinner tonight and do all the clean-up."

When I didn't say anything, he searched my face, as if looking for a clue. "I know I screwed up downstairs, and I'm truly sorry. I promise it'll never happen again."

Hot tears streamed down my face. Randy squeezed my hands and said, "I'm going to the store to get us steaks for dinner—then I'll grill them just the way you like."

I sat in that rocker for a long time, crying softly. I don't know where this thought came from, but my inner voice said, "He sounds like every other abusive man, and if you stay, you'll be like every other abused woman."

In that moment of clarity and despair, I knew I would end my marriage. Without the headache pain, I felt stronger and more confident. I wish I could say that I had the courage to end things that very day, but I didn't, even though my heart felt as if the life had been bled out of it. I couldn't respond to Randy's affection. I barely smiled or laughed when he was around. After a few days of this, he asked me, "Do you still love me?"

I hadn't felt love for him for a very long time, but I wasn't able to fully admit it to myself until the incident with the clothes. I remember looking at him and not being able to come out with anything more definitive than "I'm in an I-don't-know place."

His eyes grew wide, and his mouth hung open. "Do you still want to go on our anniversary trip?" He didn't wait for my answer. "If we don't go, we'll lose our deposit money—not that I care so much about that." I was mute. "I think we should go," Randy pleaded. "The trip can help us get back on track."

I didn't have the strength to fight him, though I knew the last thing I wanted was to spend a week alone with Randy on a romantic Caribbean island. We flew in silence to the Bahamas, only speaking to manage luggage and passports. Throughout the vacation, we didn't say much more than *hello, pass the salt,* and *what do you want to do.* There was no affection, no celebration of our twenty-five years together. I noticed that the people who worked at the resort moved away when they saw us approaching as if our sadness was contagious.

Once we got home, it took me another month or so before I told him that the marriage was over, and I was moving out of the bedroom. Randy begged me to stay in that now too-small bed. "If you move up to the guest room, we'll have to tell the kids we're getting a divorce."

I planted my feet and crossed my arms in front of me. "I just can't be in that bed with you anymore," I told him. "It's over."

He begged some more. "Can we please just go to therapy one more time? It's been a twenty-five-year-marriage. You owe me another chance."

Randy's eyes seemed to cloud with panic. Where was the man I fell so in love with at 19? His long blond hair was now combed off to the sides of his expanding bald patch and he'd long since shaved off the beard I had loved so much. He'd lost weight from all the biking and tennis, so excess skin hung on him as if he were a much older man.

Reluctantly, I agreed to go to therapy with him, but I stipulated that the therapist had to be someone neither one of us had ever worked with. We went to the first meeting together, then after that, the therapist saw each of us alone for two visits before seeing us together for his impressions.

He didn't mince any words once the hellos were out of the way. "You two don't even have anything to go back to," he said. "You've grown so far apart that you'd have to start all over."

Randy may have cried. I honestly don't remember. I know that I felt vindicated and was ready to begin taking steps to end the marriage. We talked to the kids—Eileen ran from the house sobbing, but Connor came up to me once Randy had chased after Eileen and said, "I'm happy for you, Mom. I don't know how you stood it for so long."

With the help of her therapist, Eileen eventually made peace with our decision. Randy and I decided to go to a mediator in addition to each of us engaging lawyers to help us craft an agreement. Arranging the settlement proved a very difficult and painful process to navigate, but we eventually found agreeable terms and signed the papers. I got a job teaching freshman composition courses at a local community college and moved into my own apartment in September.

And all through the separation, move, new job, and then the divorce, I was pain-free nearly every day. I felt confident that my emotional health was solid. I knew in my bones that as long as I did my part, I'd be fine. I wasn't worried about depression or the headache returning, especially since I'd gotten through the divorce and everything associated with it without a recurrence.

Since that day in May of 2000 when the migraine lifted, I've experienced brief periods of migraines—several days to a couple of weeks—but never needed anything more than one or two healing sessions with Kayla and several doses of flower essences to deal with the recurrences. The headaches serve as a flashing red light of warning that something in my life is out of balance.

Chapter 18: Why Didn't My Doctors Warn Me?

I've always wondered how I survived all of the medications I was taking—especially while under the direction of a psychiatrist and a nurse practitioner who consulted with each other and had full knowledge of my every prescription. A few years ago, alarm bells clanged in my head when media reports surfaced about the opioid epidemic devastating millions of Americans. People just like me were first treated for chronic pain with OxyContin and, later, many became addicted to heroin. Driven by the same curiosity that drove me as a child, I began investigating the use of opioids for migraines. I was shocked and angered by what I found.

In reading several online journal articles, I found that instead of decreasing pain, chronic opioid use increased pain, a phenomenon called hyperalgesia.[36] And beginning in 1943, the medical literature shows that doctors knew opioids could actually cause headaches (opioid-induced headaches) rather than cure them.[37] Even more concerning, I discovered that a condition called Medication Overuse Headache(MOH) can result from taking DHE-45, Migranol, and opioids—three of the medications I regularly used during the four years working with a headache specialist. MOH can result from using those medications for as little as ten or fifteen days or as long as three months.[38] And other researchers warned that if you are giving a daily drug with no positive results, you run the risk of harming the patient and need to consider another treatment.[39]

And here I was, taking headache medications, psychiatric drugs, and opioids—daily—for over four years. My first response to the research was disbelief. *Impossible*, I told myself. But, sadly, more and more sources confirmed what I had learned. I wondered what my nurse practitioner had known back in the 1990s when she treated me. According to a journal article I found, doctors were aware of MOH as early as the 1940s.[40] It was looking more and more like my nurse practitioner should have had at least some background knowledge about certain medications causing headaches, as well as the fact that opioids could worsen them.

Now I wonder what I was thinking and whether I had any idea of my overmedicated state. I don't think I told either doctor about my first car accident, because I saw it as a one-off event. Due to intense shame, I suppressed the whole incident. But given how shaken I was about the second accident, I'm sure I finally admitted the shambles my life had become. After that, along with the energy work, my nurse practitioner helped me to appropriately reduce the pain medications.

More reading piqued my curiosity about drug interactions, particularly the possible effects of taking Methadone and Valium together and MS-Contin or OxyContin and Valium. I found out that Methadone, invented in Germany in 1939, was found to be highly addictive. The United States approved it as a painkiller in 1947 and later used it for treating heroin withdrawal. I began taking Methadone in 1999, so with fifty-two years of history, doctors must have been aware of its effects.[41] Valium was formulated in 1963, and I began taking it in 1993. Again, the drug had a long history of use, and the doctors must have known of its dangers in combination with other sedating drugs. It didn't take me long to find many sources warning of respiratory depression and sedation, even coma and death as a result of combing them.[42]

And even though Perdue Pharma touted OxyContin as a new drug when it was released in 1996, it was simply a time-release version of Oxycodone, discovered in Germany in 1916. Again, the original drug had been on the market long enough for doctors to know of effects and dangerous interactions with other medications.[43] Yet, whenever I asked either my doctor or nurse practitioner if it was safe to take all of the drugs in combination, both of them assured me that it was. They never told me not to drive and never cautioned me about sedation and breathing problems.

The FDA warns that because women are more likely to have chronic pain, they are also more likely to be prescribed pain relievers and to use them for longer periods of time, often becoming addicted more quickly than men.[44] And I believe, along with many others, that at least part of the burden of excessive prescribing is the responsibility of Perdue Pharma's aggressive marketing campaign:

> *Because of its effectiveness and good acceptability to patients, our studies suggest that OxyContin is an ideal choice in progressive pain management when around-the-clock therapy is indicated.*
>
> *Indications and Usage: For the management of moderate to severe pain where use of an opioid analgesic is appropriate for more than a few days.* OxyContin Press Release, 1996, Purdue Pharma

I didn't know it at the time, but my doctors were practicing polypharmacy, the medical term for administering many drugs together, resulting in overmedication. Polypharmacy can increase unwanted effects or cause dangerous interactions between different drugs. As one research study concluded, "Polypharmacy often becomes a cycle of treating one condition, experiencing side effects, and treating side effects until the patient and the clinician cannot remember where the cycle began."[45]

When I tell friends about the number of drugs I was on, they shake their heads and say, "That's awful, but it wouldn't happen now." On the contrary, researchers have found that up to one third of psychiatric outpatients are on three or more psychotropic drugs. Additionally, they caution about the "growing evidence regarding the increased adverse effects—and the possibilities of cumulative toxicity and increased vulnerability to adverse events." Probably the most damning statement about medical training comes when the authors lament that even though doctors urgently need information on the "merits and demerits of polypharmacy," it has not been studied.[46]

My psychiatrist should have known better than to allow me to take so many drugs, especially Valium, along with opioids. My headache nurse should have been well-aware of the phenomenon of MOH. She, too, should have sounded an alarm over my use of a benzodiazepine and an opioid for over four years. But when those two failed in their duties to safeguard me from the potential harm of the sedating drugs I was taking, then the pharmacist should have acted as a fail-safe mechanism.

No one intervened.

Could it have been that because I appeared to be coping with my routine responsibilities, they thought I was all right? There was one person who knew I was in grave danger: my daughter. Because she spent a lot of time in the car with me, she witnessed me fall asleep at nearly every stop light. She must have been terrified. And I must have been in denial. All I know is that I felt desperate for pain relief and trusted medical personnel who worked in reputable practices to help me solve my health crisis. But it took a second car crash and an energy healer to lead me out of the nightmare that had become my life.

Chapter 19: Paradigm Shift

By the spring of 2002, even though I'd been free from depression for five years, Dr. Sherman insisted that I continue maintenance medication to ward off recurrence of depression. He told me, "You must be extra-vigilant. You've got a chemical imbalance, and your brain is damaged from repeated depressions."

At that time, my drug cocktail consisted of Wellbutrin, Valium, Elavil, and Topamax. I hardly noticed the side effects anymore, except for the dry mouth and constipation due to the Elavil. Topamax was supposed to stabilize my mood as well as help with weight loss but didn't seem very effective in helping me drop any pounds. The dose of Valium was low enough that I didn't notice any unusual sleepiness, and I was using it on an occasional basis, rather than daily. After trying innumerable antidepressants and seven rounds of ECT, I was pretty convinced that Wellbutrin was keeping me out of the dark cave of depression.

Despite my initial skepticism, I had come to believe in the chemical imbalance theory of depression. After all, I'd been well for five years thanks to the medications. At least that seemed the most plausible explanation.

But as I reflected back on all of my past experiences in seeking relief from depression, a clear picture of doctors' attitudes emerged. They didn't like to be questioned or challenged. If you were a psych patient, doctors were especially dismissive of complaints about medication-related side effects. I can remember taking Effexor and feeling hopped-up and jittery all the time, like I'd had way too much coffee to drink along with a few diet pills. My doctor at the time listened to me when I explained this problem and then said, "Well, give it a little more time. I'm sure this medication will help you."

My therapist said, "I'm sure this is the right medication for you. Just give it a few more days." So, I continued—ever mindful of the importance of being "medication-compliant." I was also desperate to find relief from the crushing depression that I felt. Effexor didn't work in a few more days or even a few more weeks, so my doctor prescribed another drug.

A year or so later, my new doctor wanted to give me Effexor. Afraid to flat-out refuse, I told him, "I took it before about a year ago, and I felt awful. Plus, it didn't work."

He listened and then handed me a prescription for Effexor, saying, "You haven't tried it with me. I know this will work." Again, desperate for relief from depression, I took it, hoping that maybe my chemical imbalance would somehow be fixed with Effexor. But I had the same response to it and moved on to yet another drug.

No matter how many I tried, none of the drugs had worked, and the darkness dragged on. I clung to the belief that depression was the result of some trauma or great difficulty in one's life— which is why people went to therapy: to untangle the web of past negative experiences, missed connections, or lost opportunities.

Then I read the 1993 edition of *Listening to Prozac* by Peter Kramer. Kramer's writing was so compelling that his book served as the linchpin to convince me that depression was caused by a deficit of the neurotransmitters serotonin or norepinephrine, or, in some cases, a combination of the two.

Despite my initial wariness about the chemical imbalance explanation early in my treatment, I was persuaded because my doctors and therapists used the same line of reasoning to convince me to take medication: comparing depression to diabetes—both of them chronic. The prevailing wisdom held that depression was hereditary, like my blue eyes and curly hair—from my dad. And here was the other gift of heredity—depression from my mom.

When it came to finding out about the drugs I was taking, I wasn't following directions blindly. I read as much as I could get my hands on about psychiatric medications and their side effects, and, at the time, the most comprehensive source of information on all drugs (written for laypeople) was a publication called *The Pill Book*, written by a pharmacist. I was intent on reading about the possible side effects of the drugs I was taking, so I could monitor myself to see what the source of any unusual reactions might be. But like most people, I trusted the FDA and the drug approval process to be above reproach, and I certainly trusted my doctors to be ethical. So, if they all said that the drugs were safe and effective for most people, I believed them.

But all of that was about to change in the spring of 2002 when I read some of my University of Maryland students' research papers. Two research papers, written by pre-nursing students, piqued my curiosity with their claims about the potential harm that could come from taking psychotropic medications, the over-prescription of Selective Serotonin/Norepinephrine Reuptake Inhibitors (SSRIs or SSNRIs), and lax or even fraudulent research practices during the clinical trials. The names of the drugs read like a long list of things that had all been in my medicine cabinet—Prozac, Zoloft, Paxil, Effexor, Wellbutrin, and Serzone.

One of their sources that appeared repeatedly was *Prozac Backlash*, written in 2000 by Joseph Glenmullen, a Harvard Medical School faculty member and practicing psychiatrist. Lucky for me, my county library had a copy. He opened the book with diagrams and descriptions of how the psychiatric drugs work. The term "Selective Serotonin Reuptake Inhibitor" had previously sounded too complex for me to understand. But now that I was pain-free, I could take the time to investigate how the drugs worked and what effect they could have on my brain.

And this information was vitally important for me to

understand—because for the past nine years, I'd had a bunch of doctors insisting that depression was caused by a lack of serotonin in the brain. Easy to fix, they had all promised. Just find the right drug and the right dose, take the drug forever, and no more depression. Glenmullen's thoughtful use of research revealed an entirely different story.

His diagrams illustrated how neurotransmitters communicate with each other. He explained that when more serotonin than normal stays in the synapses (gaps between the nerve endings), other neurotransmitters are also affected. For example, he said that doctors are discovering that when serotonin is increased, dopamine—the "feel-good" neurotransmitter—is decreased. He went on to explain how lowered levels of dopamine can be responsible for some of the more severe side effects of the Prozac-type drugs, effects that he calls "Prozac Backlash," which includes facial tics, inner-agitation, muscle spasms, and drug-induced parkinsonism. He concluded by saying, "The unfortunate irony is that drugs heavily promoted as correcting unproven biochemical imbalances may, in fact, be causing imbalances and brain damage."[47]

I was already feeling upset, and I had only read the introduction. *How could this be? Why didn't I know this stuff? Why hadn't any doctors told me?* Whenever I asked doctors about side effects or long-term use, they told me that the drugs were perfectly safe and that the side effects only happened to a few people. But now I was thinking *What if I'm one of those few?* The news did not get better.

Glenmullen explained how clinical trials work and that the researchers are only required to show that drugs are effective in the relatively short period of six to eight weeks, despite the fact that "…serious side effects of drugs take years, sometimes decades to emerge. Under these circumstances, prescribing an entirely new class of agents to millions of people is nothing short of ongoing human experimentation."[48] *Great, I've been taking Wellbutrin and Topamax for over five years, and even the even drug companies don't know what their meds could do to me.*

Another effect of the Prozac-like drugs is what doctors refer to as *neurologically driven agitation*. Glenmullen described one of his patients who felt like he had "coffee running in his veins" and who literally couldn't stop pacing during the day and moving about restlessly in his bed at night. Other patients reported feeling as if their heads were going to explode, and with those two examples, I knew I'd found the answer to the problem of why I felt so awful on Effexor.

I remember telling the doctor that I felt like I was going to jump out of my skin. Nevertheless, my doctor insisted that I stay on the drug for the full six weeks to give it a fair try. Now I had confirmation of what I'd experienced. Not only that, but psychiatric research had documented that neurologically driven agitation was a common side-effect for between 10 to 25 percent of patients taking the Prozac-like drugs or SSRIs. Shouldn't my doctor have known that?

And along with the imbalance in serotonin and dopamine comes the phenomenon of what doctors euphemistically call "Prozac poop-out," where a drug that formerly provided relief from symptoms of depression no longer works, despite higher and higher doses. Or, in some cases, patients go off the drugs, and then when they restart due to withdrawal symptoms that mimic depression, the drug no longer works. In reality, the brain is compensating for the drug-induced changes.

Wow, I was only on page fifty and felt like I'd learned all I needed to know to get off the drugs. Even though I no longer took Prozac, Effexor, Zoloft, or Paxil, I knew from my doctor that Wellbutrin was a close cousin to all of them, and I wasn't going to wait another ten years to find out if that drug did the same thing. I felt the sharp twist in the pit of my stomach. *Why did it take a book to tell me the truth? Weren't my doctors reading medical journals and going to conferences?*

And when I read about one effect of the drugs, I realized it was already too late for someone I loved—my mother. As soon as I read Glenmullen's description of tardive dyskenisia (abnormal movements), I recognized something that my mother had been doing for a long time—tongue-darting. My mother, who'd taken all kinds of psychiatric drugs for over thirty years, would often stick her tongue way out of her mouth almost as if she were gagging and then pull it back in. I hated to see her doing this, but at least now I knew why. But there are other tics, or involuntary movements that can happen, including what the shrinks call "chewing the cud" and facial tics, like twitching of the eyes. These side effects show up only after the clinical trials are over. And for many patients, they can be permanent.[49] Like in my mother's case.

One day when I was visiting Mom in the nursing home, she was seized with full-body shaking that wouldn't let up. That afternoon, Mom sat in her wheelchair and greeted me with a smile the way she always did. But after a minute or so, I noticed that she was trembling uncontrollably. "Mom, what's wrong? Do you have a fever?" I felt her forehead, but her temperature seemed normal.

"Ann, I can't stop shaking. It's been going on all day."

I was alarmed by her appearance and very concerned, because I could sense her deep distress. I'd seen Mom shake before, but never so irrepressibly and never for more than an hour or so. "Have you called a nurse to come and help you? Do you want me to call Dr. C.?" (her general practitioner, whose office was next door to the nursing home).

"No, I don't want to bother anyone. I hope it will stop soon. Just stay with me and talk," she said. Her eyes searched my face, and she squeezed both of my hands.

We sat across from each other and talked for a few minutes, but the tremors worsened. Instinctively, I stood behind Mom and wrapped my arms around her in a tight hug.

"Thank you, honey," was all she said.

But the shaking intensified. I had no idea what to do, but I knew something was terribly wrong.

"Do you want me to call your doctor, Mom?"

"I'm not sure. Maybe this will pass."

Typical of Mom to refuse to call any attention to herself. But as I stood behind her and felt her small body tremble incessantly, I decided to do something. I wheeled Mom down the hall and parked her in front of the nurses' station. The charge nurse, Betty, looked up and asked if she could help.

"I sure hope so," I said. "My mother can't stop shaking, and it's been going on all day. She didn't want to bother anyone, but I decided that the situation is unacceptable. I'm not leaving until you call her doctor and get this resolved."

Betty's face didn't change. "I'm not sure what we can do, Ms. Dempsey. The doctor isn't due for a visit today."

I continued wrapping my mother in a bear-hug as she shook. I felt my jaw muscles tighten as we waited in the hallway, and I struggled to cover my annoyance.

"Look, this is an emergency. Dr. C. is next door, and I'm pretty sure this situation has something to do with Mom's meds. Look at her!" I demanded. "You know this shaking isn't right. Call the doctor, please."

Betty sat back down and looked in Mom's chart.

"I'm not leaving until someone helps my mother."

By now, other staff had heard some of the conversation. I was creating a scene, but I thought it was the only way to get immediate help. After what seemed like hours, Betty finally called Dr. C. and told her about Mom's condition—and that I had Mom in the hallway and wouldn't move until the doctor took action.

A few minutes later, Dr. C. burst through the swinging doors, glanced at Mom's chart, then locked eyes with me. "What are you so concerned about, Ms. Dempsey? Your mother isn't on any new medications, so I'm not sure what the problem is." She faced us and folded her arms across her chest.

"I'm not sure either, doctor, but I know something's terribly wrong, and it's probably related to Mom's medications. Like I told the nurse, I'm not leaving here until you do something to help my mother." All the while, I had my arms wrapped around Mom who said nothing but continued to tremble.

I don't know how long we faced-off in the hallway, staring each other down, but after reviewing Mom's chart and talking with Betty out of earshot, Dr. C. had an answer.

"Ms. Dempsey, I'm going to take care of this situation, but I'm not doing it for your mother or your father. I'm doing it to get you off my back." Dr. C. planted her feet and crossed her arms tightly across her chest.

"I don't care why you help her, I just care that you do something. I've never seen Mom like this, and she's very upset. To leave her shaking uncontrollably is unacceptable, and I'm glad you decided to do the right thing."

After that day, I don't remember Mom having non-stop, whole-body tremors ever again. She didn't go to the hospital, and I don't know what Dr. C. did to control the shaking. But thanks to finding Dad's records, I've been able to piece together the likely pharmaceutical culprits for the damage that occurred years earlier.

I was shocked to see that Mom had taken Thorazine for a number of years—a drug which I'd always associated with people who were schizophrenic. I didn't know much at all about the drug, just that it zoned people out and was a heavy-duty sedative. An old friend of mine used to talk about her clients who took the drug as doing the "Thorazine shuffle," because they were too zombified to pick up their feet when they walked. But once I began digging into the literature and looking at drug ads from the fifties and sixties, a different picture emerged.

Thorazine, classified as both a major tranquilizer and a neuroleptic, was widely prescribed for all kinds of "maladies" and conditions after it came into use in the early fifties. In fact, doctors used the drug for problems as varied as nausea, pain, and behavior problems in children. Because Thorazine rendered patients quiet and passive, some doctors likened its effects as being equivalent to a chemical lobotomy, rendering patients "lethargic, disinterested, and childlike," a state considered to be an improvement over patients who were anxious and agitated or having psychotic thoughts. One skeptical doctor, E. H. Parsons, cautioned in 1955 that the use of Thorazine was not treating an actual pathology of the mind, but rather it was used "to produce specific effect."[50]

In addition, beginning in the early 1960s, numerous reports emerged about patients having issues with tardive dyskinesia (tics), muscle spasms, parkinsonism, and agitation. To counteract those effects, many doctors prescribed Cogentin, which Mom took during her first hospitalization in 1959. Dad's notes say that the drug "upset her," and I only see it listed once in the records.

The reports of tics continued to mount through the sixties and seventies, but the FDA took no action to place warnings on the drug until 1985, almost thirty years after it had been introduced. By then, millions of people worldwide had used the drug for conditions as common as nausea and gastrointestinal distress or simply to maintain quiet and order in psychiatric wards. Dad's records indicate that Mom took Thorazine and several other major tranquilizers for over seventeen years and antidepressants for over thirty years—both of which can cause full-body tremors.

Chapter 20: What Could a Patient Possibly Understand About Clinical Trials?

Glenmullen's book opened my eyes to the realities of clinical trials and how the profit incentive can overshadow ethics when it comes to drug approval. He describes how prior to Prozac's approval in 1988, most antidepressants were prescribed by psychiatrists and required frequent monitoring for side effects and dosage increases. But in the 1970s and eighties, primary care doctors had begun to prescribe psychiatric drugs and were uncomfortable with the complex and frequent monitoring required for tricyclics—the class of early antidepressants. In response, Eli Lilly developed Prozac in a twenty-milligram dose to work for everyone, requiring only twice-yearly monitoring—a schedule that suited general practitioners' desire to have a drug that was easy to administer.

Very early on after Prozac's initial release to the general public, doctors were requesting that Eli Lilly create five- and ten-milligram doses for those patients who had great difficulty dealing with the anxiety and agitation associated with taking Prozac. Lilly had heard similar complaints as early as 1979 when Dr. Ray Fuller, one of the doctors responsible for inventing Prozac, reported that "...some patients have converted from severe depression to agitation within a few days.... In future studies, the use of benzodiazepines (Valium-type sedatives) to control agitation will be permitted." Glenmullen goes on to say that Lilly's protocols allowed for researchers to prescribe sedatives—which served to mask the side effects—for any patient who became anxious, agitated, or sleepless.

And even though drug companies were shown repeated cases of harmful side effects, they usually defended their drugs no matter what the consequences to the patient.[51]

From a patient's perspective, I found this information very disturbing. I thought back on all of the drugs that I had tried, especially Effexor, that had caused me to feel extremely agitated. I remembered begging one of the doctors to take me off the drug, yet he kept me on Effexor another week or more to see if it would work—completely dismissing my concerns. I began to wonder if the near-crippling anxiety I'd suffered was actually a part of my depression or caused by the meds that were supposed to be helping me.

According to Glenmullen, Lilly did not recommend sedatives in the prescribing guidelines for fear of complicating the one-size-fits-all model—even though they were used in the clinical trials. Based on what I'd learned about trials in grad school, I knew that using one drug to mask the effects of another was not the right way to run an experiment. Dr. Nancy Lord, an authority on testing new drugs for FDA approval, described the practice of using sedatives while testing an antidepressant as improper. She stated that allowing other drugs in the trials that acted on the brain "completely obscured what this product [Prozac] was doing to people's minds."[52]

But the worst information that Glenmullen revealed was about the many patients who participated in the clinical trials had feelings of wanting to commit suicide, often referred to as suicidal ideation. Suicidal thoughts were routinely labeled or coded in the databases as "depression." In other words, the side effect of wanting to commit suicide was simply labeled as the problem for which the patient was seeking treatment.

Dr. Lord described the trials as "worthless" due to the practices that Lilly had engaged in. But for me, the final nail in Prozac's coffin was that the German researchers wouldn't approve the drug because of the increases in agitation, suicidal ideation, and the use of sedatives to mask both side effects. Glenmullen stated that he and other psychiatrists had witnessed similar effects of the drug in their patients—within weeks of starting Prozac, patients often reported feeling outside of themselves and having thoughts of suicide and violence, and even edged toward psychosis.[53]

I could hardly wait for my next appointment with my therapist, Pauline. The information I was reading was deeply upsetting, and I wanted to talk with her about coming off of my awful drug cocktail. I'd been depression-free since 1997—five years—and now I was more afraid of the drugs than I was of another depression. I knew Dr. Sherman wouldn't approve, but after reading just a few chapters in Glenmullen's book, I was determined to stop taking the drugs. I hoped that Pauline wouldn't dismiss my concerns the way that previous doctors and therapists had.

I couldn't put *Prozac Backlash* down. What would the research reveal about Wellbutrin and Topamax? Both drugs were relatively new and certainly newer than the Prozac-like drugs. I had read voraciously all during my depression, trying to find some explanation that made sense. In retrospect, *Listening to Prozac* by Peter Kramer seemed like a gigantic lie, yet all of my doctors had recommended that I read it. "You have a chemical imbalance," they'd told me. "The meds are safe, and you'll need to take them for the rest of your life." Now more than ever, I wasn't so sure.

Chapter 21: You Have a Damaged Brain

I began referencing *Prozac Backlash* during my appointments with Pauline, until one day I announced, "I'm coming off of these drugs. There doesn't seem to be enough research about their long-term effects, and I'm not willing to be a Guinea pig any longer." After discussing the best way to begin tapering my antidepressants and Valium, we decided to start with Topamax, a mood stabilizer, since it was the last drug added to my cocktail, and the one that had been in my system for the least amount of time. In my mind, that was the drug that I least needed since I no longer believed that I had what the Hopkins doctor had called "mild, atypical hypomania" or what Dr. Sherman casually referred to as Bipolar II.

Pauline didn't see me as fitting that diagnosis either.

"I've worked with you for three years now—since 1999—and I've never seen you having any extreme mood swings. In fact, you've navigated your divorce, move, and full-time job very successfully. I think you're a good candidate to taper off of your meds."

Because she worked in a state mental health facility, Pauline seemed to know quite a bit about tapering safely. And while she urged me to talk with Dr. Sherman, I refused. "I'm sick of doctors at this point, and I don't want to deal with him if he tries to scare me into staying on the drugs. It's my body. Don't I have a right to do what I want?"

"Of course, you do, Ann. Every patient has the absolute right to question a doctor about medications and even to refuse them if they don't like the side effects or feel they want to try life without drugs."

Because Pauline and I had been working together in therapy for a few years, I felt that she knew me very well. I was comfortable talking to her, and we had a lot in common, including our love of poetry. In addition, though we didn't always use poetry to frame our sessions, Pauline was trained as a poetry therapist and believed very much as I did in the power of metaphor and myth to tap into realms that linear thought couldn't untangle. I was going through poetry therapy training at the time as well and had done a lot of reading on psychology, group process, and the role of the arts in healing.

We talked about all of the doctors that I'd seen and how they'd tried numerous medications in an attempt to get my feelings of depression under control. Before it finally lifted, I frequently complained to Dr. Sherman about taking so many medications, often saying that I felt like a chemical waste dump.

I was glad to be off the headache drugs, and I felt so much more alive and competent. Now I just had to get off the psych meds, starting with Topamax. I don't remember how many milligrams I took, but I recall cutting the pills into smaller and smaller increments—first halving the dose, then trying a quarter, and finally moving to every other day with an eighth of a pill. Because I had no problems at all coming off of that drug, we moved on to the Wellbutrin.

It's important to note here that tapering off of any medication is a highly individualized process. In 2002 when I was discontinuing my medications, there were virtually no resources to advise people. Now, there are numerous online resources, including The Inner Compass Initiative's Withdrawal Project and Surviving Antidepressants, just to name a couple. From what I've read, I was very fortunate that my withdrawal from psych drugs was relatively seamless.

Here is where I lose the details—I don't remember exactly what I did to taper, but I probably asked Dr. Sherman for a lower dose just to try it out, and then reduced my dose even more over time by cutting the pills into smaller and smaller pieces. Ever since I'd had a complete recovery, he'd been adamant about my needing to take antidepressants forever. "Your brain has been damaged with each successive episode of depression," he'd tell me. "Odds are that if you stop taking your meds, you'll have an even worse depression than the one you just kicked."

Prior to reading Glenmullen's book and seeing all of the studies that my students cited in their papers, I'd placed complete trust in Dr. Sherman. I'm sure some transference was operating since he'd helped me when no one else could. And he'd supported me in getting out of my marriage. As far as I was concerned, he was a good guy. But my faith was waning now that I'd done some deeper investigating.

Pauline and I kept close tabs on how I was feeling throughout the tapering process, and I seemed to be doing fine. I know it took me several months to get off of the Wellbutrin and Topamax. That left two drugs to go: Valium and Elavil. Any anxiety that I felt was transient and often related to job-challenges, so I only used the Valium on an as-needed basis. According to my records, I took about five milligrams a day if needed. Plus, I had Kava Kava, an herbal supplement and my work-around when it came to managing anxiety and using less Valium.

I remember how I started using Kava Kava—when the dose of Valium wore off, I could feel the anxiety clamp down on me, like hands squeezing around my throat. For several years when I was depressed, I remember rolling out of bed in the morning and taking a Valium before I did anything else. I was miserable, frightened, and desperate to find a better way to deal with the awful daily terrors that greeted me every morning.

Either a friend mentioned Kava Kava or I'd read about it, so I began taking it sometimes instead of my next dose of Valium. What I remember loving about the supplement was that I didn't have the awful seizing feelings anymore; I just felt calm and relaxed all day.

And now that I was living on my own and working as a teacher, I felt less and less anxiety, so taking five milligrams of Valium on a few-times-a-week basis didn't seem like much of an issue to me. After all, for over seven years, my doctors had routinely dosed me with Valium and other benzodiazepines to tamp down my feelings of anxiety.

Instead, they should have followed the prescribing guidelines that I discovered in the 1998 edition of *The Pill Book*. Those guidelines cautioned that Valium shouldn't be taken beyond three to four months and that prescribers should avoid giving it to patients with severe depression. Currently, only short-term use—two to four weeks— of benzodiazepines is recommended. After that, patients benefit more from therapy and treatments that teach them how to manage stress, breathing to induce calming feelings, and the use of herbal teas and exercise. Instead of actively prescribing Valium for years and telling me it was safe, my therapists and doctors should have known this information and worked to help me deal with anxiety differently.

In 2021, the United States Food and Drug Administration (FDA) issued a statement "requiring class-wide labeling changes for benzodiazepines [like Valium, Klonopin, and Xanax)… to help improve their safe use." When I was taking Valium, no ever warned me of any of these problems. In the 2021 statement, FDA Commissioner Stephen M. Hahn, M.D. said, "We are taking measures and requiring new labeling information to help health care professionals and patients better understand that while benzodiazepines have many treatment benefits, they also carry with them an increased risk of abuse, misuse, addiction and dependence." I wish my doctors and therapists had offered me some information about the dangers of Valium instead of treating it like a sugar pill.

But I was even more eager to get off of Elavil. I'd been on it since 1994, and it was now 2002, so that was eight years of the little red pill's chemicals circulating through my body. I was tired of the dry mouth and the deep, dark sleep that it induced. And the constipation, necessitating prunes and even Sennakot pills to have some sense of regularity. Since I'd taken Elavil twice before and successfully gotten off of it, I anticipated the same would be true this time. I was only taking fifteen milligrams (or some very small dose, I don't remember exactly) at night, which is a very low dose, so I began by cutting it in half. No problem. I did that for a few weeks and then went to a quarter for a few weeks. No problem. Then an eighth, and finally I stopped taking it all together. *Woo hoo!* I was home free, I thought. Then WHAM—my migraine roared back with incredible force, and I panicked.

"How can this be? I haven't had a migraine in over two years, and suddenly it's back again?" I wailed to Pauline. I was spooked and began taking the Elavil again. "I can't work as long as I have a headache, and I sure as heck need to work."

"Ann, calm down. You'll be fine. The little bit of Elavil that you're taking is probably just what you need to keep all systems in gear," Pauline assured me. "Besides, now you're off of all headache meds and two of your psych meds. I'd say you're in great shape!"

I listened to Pauline's wisdom, mostly because I was terrified of the migraine's return. I decided to wait until summer when I didn't have to teach to try again with dumping Elavil and finally being drug-free. Still, I was unsuccessful, so I stayed on that darn drug.

A few years later after several failed attempts, I found a web-based support group for people struggling to stop Elavil. What a revelation to learn that headaches were a frequent effect of discontinuing the drug and could be helped by taking supplements and slowing the taper even more. I decided to try once more, and within a few months, I was completely off and haven't used it since then.

But my experience looks like a picnic compared to some of the information I've discovered about discontinuing psychiatric drugs. Psychologist Laysah Ostrow published the results of her 2017 study on discontinuing antidepressants in the journal *Psychiatric Services*. Patients in the study, who had been taking medications between nine months and nine years, took a wide variety of psychiatric drugs, including anxiolytics, antidepressants, antipsychotics, mood stabilizers, and stimulants, and all of them were attempting to discontinue one or two prescriptions. The three main reasons for wanting to discontinue the drugs included concerns about long-term effects, adverse side effects, and feeling like the drugs prevented them from self-understanding.

The study participants described a very difficult discontinuation experience and noted sleep disturbance, increased anxiety, sadness and tearfulness, fatigue, flu-like symptoms, and "brain zaps" or neurological problems. Additionally, they said the best sources of help were "family, friends, and self-care practices," but, sadly, not their mental health providers.[54]

All the while that I was tapering off of Wellbutrin, Topamax, and Elavil, I'd been seeing Dr. Sherman every two months for medication checks and never told him what I was doing. It never occurred to me that I was behaving exactly the way my father had behaved with my mother's doctors. I was lying—at least by omitting the truth of what I was doing.

We'd had lots of discussions in the past where I'd challenged Dr. Sherman on his insistence that I had Bipolar II and needed a mood stabilizer. "If the medications cause a condition, then the condition is a side-effect, not a real illness," I'd said to him.

Dr. Sherman was always very relaxed and informal, taking my minor objections in stride. He never seemed to get riled up about anything; in fact, he didn't even sit up straight in his arm chair like most doctors. Instead, he slouched way down in the seat, stuck his chubby legs out in front of him, and propped my chart on the shelf of his belly. He'd peer over his glasses and say, "Ann, I'm convinced everyone is at least a little bipolar. Besides, if you're functioning well on all of your meds, why rock the boat?" And for several years, I had gone along with his recommendation. But now that I done some serious reading, I was skeptical. I made an appointment and went to tell him that I was off of my meds and wasn't coming back.

I took *Prozac Backlash* to my appointment so I could refer to specific sections that I'd marked. I knew that I wanted to discuss the corrupt clinical trials and the fact that antidepressants, not depression, change the chemical functioning of the brain. And as long as I could cite actual studies, I was sure that Dr. Sherman would have to agree that the *evidence* was solid, even if he didn't buy the premise. Maybe he'd even read some of the same studies in his psychiatry journals. He knew that I was a voracious reader and did lots of research on any topic that interested me, and nothing interested me more now than information about the dangers of psychiatric medications. Especially since I'd seen what they'd done to my mother after her forty or more years of use. I was prepared for some pushback, but I had complete faith that eventually Dr. Sherman would see it my way.

He lounged in his chair as I entered the office. His desk was piled high with newspapers, and file folders tumbled out from under end-tables, while a pile of journals teetered on the edge of the shelf. His Civil War sword stood guard on top of a bookshelf, and a large photograph of MLK looked down on the mess of an office. Why was I noticing all of the clutter? I knew it had been there before, but it looked much worse today. I was kind of nervous, but I jumped in with a teaser.

"Bet you can't guess what I've just done."

"Murdered your ex with a baseball bat?"

We both laughed.

"No, but I keep one ready in case I need to get a message through to him."

Dr. Sherman waited, hands folded on his bulging stomach, sleeves rolled up revealing white, fleshy arms. He'd suffered a heart attack a few years back and had lost weight right after, but it looked like the pounds were creeping back up.

"Well, my students have been doing some interesting papers on over-prescription of antidepressants," I began, flipping a few pages of the Glenmullen book.

He smiled.

"I've learned some things that make me question taking psych meds—at least now that I've been depression-free for five years." Dr. Sherman peered over his glasses and looked at me.

"So, you're taking some ideas from student papers over what I've been telling you all this time?"

"No, of course not. When I first read all of the claims they were making, I thought they were over-reacting."

Dr. Sherman just looked at me. "And so…"

"But after I'd read several of their papers and took a look at some of the research they were citing, I decided to find one of the books they'd used." I hadn't expected resistance so early on. Dr. Sherman peered at me over his glasses. His slumped posture never shifted while I fidgeted a little in my chair, formulating my next foray. *Where do I go now?*

"Well, one thing I wanted to ask you about was the evidence I discovered about the clinical trials of Prozac." Dr. Sherman looked at me and waited. I held up Glenmullen's book. "Ever heard of him?"

"No."

I swallowed and put the book down. "He's a psychiatrist who teaches at Harvard Medical School, and he has a practice in Boston. I'm surprised you don't know about him."

"He's not somebody who's on my radar. And you know I do clinical trials myself," he said.

"Yeah, I know. All the more reason I thought you might be familiar with his work. Anyway, what Glenmullen says about Prozac's clinical trials is really disturbing."

He had to listen. Why didn't Dr. Sherman know any of this stuff?

"You're not on Prozac, Ann. Besides, I've used the drug for years with patients and many of them do quite well. What's got you so upset?"

My stomach clenched. His tone was abrupt and dismissive, just like my father when I stood up to him. Just like Randy when he didn't want to hear what I had to say. But Dr. Sherman had never spoken to me like this before. I also told him about the German investigators refusing to continue the trials due to the increased risk of suicide attempts. I told him about the concern about the addition of Valium to the trial.[55]

Dr. Sherman nodded. "So? Maybe they were a little energized after being depressed for so long. Prozac's a good drug and it's been around for over ten years now…"

I asked him about the suicides and then reminded him that the description I'd read about Effexor was exactly the way I'd felt—like I was going to jump out of my skin. I told him about the research I'd read that concluded some people got so agitated that they committed suicide even though they were never suicidal to begin with. I thumbed through my book. *Why hadn't I marked that page?*

Dr. Sherman began fidgeting with my file and drumming his fingers, but still slumped in his chair. His tone changed from one of humor to defensive bordering on arrogant. "I don't know where this Glenmullen guy got the research that's in that book, but I can tell you I've never read any of that stuff, and I trust what I've seen with Prozac helping my patients. Leave the research to me. You stick to teaching poetry."

I felt like he'd slammed a door in my face, so I took another hallway and asked him about the short window of testing and the fact that no research was done on long-term side effects, which often take years to show up.

"Ann, first of all, you're not on Prozac. And second, you're not having any problems with side effects now that we've got you on Wellbutrin and Topamax," he said.

"That's not the point," I said. "I've seen the side effects in my mother, and she's never taken Prozac. She has tardive dyskenisia, and she does this awful thing with her tongue that she can't control."

Dr. Sherman shrugged. "I've seen that in some older folks," was all he offered. Then he looked at his watch—a rare occurrence.

I was done with trying to show him what I'd learned. Time to tell him about my decision.

"Well, I'm not willing to see if anything bad happens to my brain. I've already stopped taking Wellbutrin and Topamax, and I feel fine. Valium, I keep around just in case, but I'm not taking it on a daily basis. It's been a couple of months already."

Dr. Sherman peered at me and sat up a little in his chair. His face softened. "Ann, you've been through an awful depression. You have a damaged brain, and if you stay off of these drugs, your depression will come back worse than you can even imagine. I care about you, and I don't want to see that happen."

A damaged brain? That was the best he could do? I leaned toward him. "Well, it's my body and my life. I'm not willing to take a chance with injury that could show up years from now. Besides, I've been depression-free for five years now. I've started a new career, bought a house, started dating again…"

"Yes, you've done well. And you've been on meds the whole time."

"I know, but now I have new information, and I'm making a new decision. If I get depressed again, maybe I'll take the meds. But for now, it's my body, and I'm not willing to experiment anymore."

Dr. Sherman stared at me for a few seconds, then shrugged. "Suit yourself, but don't say I didn't warn you. As for me, I'm never giving up my Prozac and Xanax, even if they've completely destroyed my libido."

I looked at him with fresh eyes. And sadness. The person who'd been my rock, the person that I credited with saving me from depression—this person was just another human.

Chapter 22: The Book of Revelation

One day in 2011, my daughter Eileen called me, sobbing into the phone. "Mom, I don't know what to do. I feel an awful blackness again, and I'm having thoughts of killing myself."

Eileen had recently transferred from teaching at a high school to a high-needs middle school and was working long hours nearly every day. "It's like my first year of teaching all over again," she cried into the phone. "All I do is work."

She detailed all of the original lessons she had to create and the challenges of adjusting to a new faculty and administration.

"I've never worked with middle school kids before, and they can be awful to deal with sometimes."

I knew that she struggled to manage her classes of thirty-plus students who often misbehaved and needed a lot of her patience and attention.

"And now when I'm driving, I get these images of crashing into trees. Mom, I don't want to hurt myself, and I keep remembering before when I was cutting."

I gripped the phone and fought my first impulse, which was to tell her she'd be OK if she could just ride things out. I worried that she didn't have the emotional strength to cope with the dark thoughts and the feelings of being overwhelmed that came with taking on a new teaching job. "Have you called Maria? She's helped you before, and maybe she can recommend a good psychiatrist."

Eileen managed to see her therapist almost immediately and then got a referral for a female psychiatrist who put her on Wellbutrin, the antidepressant she'd used in the past. When we spoke a few days later, she seemed calmer and more in control.

"Mom, the doctor said since the Wellbutrin worked before, it will probably work again. I'm already feeling better and more hopeful."

I had two reactions: my Mom-self wanted to protect my daughter and keep her out of all pain. My adult-self knew that Eileen needed therapy to address the way she saw herself both at work and on a personal level. "I believe that, too, Eileen. Will you be seeing Maria soon?"

"Yeah, I have an appointment in a few days. Maria's always so helpful."

Just be quiet, I told myself. *Now is not the time to caution her about taking medication.* Based on my history of maintaining a steady emotional state once I'd gotten out of my marriage, I had a lot of questions about the whole chemical imbalance theory. So, I did what I always do when I'm curious about a topic—went online and researched more books on antidepressants.

All sorts of titles popped up, but the most intriguing one was *The Anatomy of an Epidemic: Magic Bullets, Psychiatric Drugs, and the Astonishing Rise of Mental Illness in America* by Robert Whitaker. There was a link to purchase the book on Amazon, so I clicked and began to "search inside this book." I was intrigued by the reviews, which confirmed some of my misgivings about the drugs. Whitaker's work appeared to build on ideas I'd first read in *Prozac Backlash*—both he and Glenmullen were challenging the notion that depression is the result of a chemical imbalance in the brain and should be treated with antidepressants. Of course, I had inklings of the same idea, but here was an investigative reporter digging into the research. And just in time for my daughter to possibly take an alternative path to wellness.

Whitaker's book arrived a few days later, and I began reading immediately. One of the early psychiatric drugs he discussed was Miltown, developed in 1955. "Take your Miltown," Dad used to say when Mom became very upset or agitated. It was known as a minor tranquilizer, capable of calming anxiety in both animals and humans. But more than just calming people, the drug produced a numbed-out state, which I remembered in my mother. One reporter in *Science News* explained the effects of Miltown this way: "If you took a minor tranquilizer (Miltown and Librium) this would mean that you could still feel scared when you see a car speeding toward you, but the fear would not make you run."[56] Now Mom's extreme passivity made sense—the way she just agreed to everything and didn't put up a fight or challenge my father. My body flooded with anger as I thought about my mother and the thousands of other people, mostly women, who had been given drugs to render them numb and passive.

As I read about the early history of psychiatric drugs, I thought back to when I was a little girl. When I observed my mother, I saw a person who was sick and who took medicine to get better. But she never "got better" for more than a few days to a week before sliding back into either a tearful, anxious state or a very fatigued state where it almost seemed like her feet were weighted with lead. When Dad would send us off to bed, he'd admonish us to "Pray for your mother to get well." So, very early on the seed was planted in my heart and mind that one day Mom would recover and be the happy, active person she was before she became depressed. The medicines never made her well—a fact that made me question the whole chemical imbalance theory, especially now that I was reading *The Anatomy of an Epidemic*. But I also knew from watching Mom, reading about mental illness, and talking with my doctors and therapists that Mom's drinking contributed to her inability to get well.

I had recovered from a severe depression—due to meds? ECT? time? poetry? therapy? I'm still not sure, but I know that poetry made more sense of my emotional state than any other kind of intervention. Contrary to Dr. Sherman's dire warning, I didn't seem to have a damaged brain, and that "worse than you've ever had" depression hadn't materialized. I'd stayed well now for nine years without the "help" of any psychiatric drugs since tapering off of them. I had plenty of reasons to doubt the chemical imbalance theory, so I kept reading.

Given some of the awful side effects of the drugs, I wondered why doctors had been so intent on finding a magic pill to help people with emotional distress. The best answer I could come up with was that many researchers were motivated by a sincere desire to relieve people suffering from mental anguish. From my own experience, I knew that therapy could take a very long time to unravel any cause for depression and many people either didn't have the time, the desire, or the money to pursue therapy. I remember my father saying that Mom would often go to see her psychiatrist—back when they did therapy—and never talked. I couldn't understand why at the time, but I've come to understand the very patriarchal nature of medicine that probably kept Mom from sharing her deepest feelings. And finally, many people just want to feel better and doctors were trained to alleviate pain, so the hunt for the "magic pill" made sense.

My doctors, therapists, and many books and articles that I had read all told the same simple story of what caused depression. While all of those sources acknowledged that stressful life events might result in depression (situational depression), many times the illness was deemed hereditary and caused by a chemical imbalance in the brain (clinical depression). However, the *treatment* for the two distinct types of depression usually remained the same: medication with therapy. But what about people like me who tried numerous meds and ECT before ever feeling better? Nowadays, many doctors would label my predicament as "treatment-resistant" depression and recommend ECT.

According to the doctors researching antidepressants, they believed that the chemical imbalance was either in serotonin and/or norepinephrine for depression or dopamine for schizophrenia. Pretty specific targeting for a system as complex as the human brain, which contains roughly 150 trillion synapses. Clearly, it's an extraordinarily complex system, so how did doctors pinpoint exactly what neurotransmitters were implicated in depression?[57]

Doctors and scientific researchers formed the chemical imbalance theory after looking at the effects of the drugs on the brain chemistry of rats, rabbits, and other mammals and then reasoned backwards. They theorized that if a drug increased certain levels of neurotransmitters, then depression must be a result of a lack of that chemical.

Of course, as a patient and a layperson, I had no idea of any of this information about the research behind the chemical imbalance theory of depression. Doctors told my father that my mother had a chemical imbalance, and thirty years later they told me the same story. I was amazed to discover all of this research on a topic that had always been presented to me as scientific fact. In his book *Depression Delusion*, Terry Lynch, Irish psychotherapist and medical doctor, included pages of research and notes from psychiatrists who debunked the "chemical imbalance" theory with strong and unambiguous language:

> *"...there is no convincing evidence that most mental patients have any chemical imbalance. Yet many physicians tell their patients they are suffering from a chemical imbalance despite the reality that there are no tests available for assessing the chemical status of a living person's brain."*
> ~Elliott Valenstein, 1998, author of Blaming the Brain

> *"It is now widely assumed that our serotonin levels fall when we feel low...but there is no evidence for any of this, nor has there ever been...No abnormality of serotonin in depression has ever been demonstrated."*
> ~David Healy, 2006, author of Let Them Eat Prozac: The Unhealthy Relationship Between the Pharmaceutical Industry and Depression

Terry Lynch also quotes Stanford psychiatrist David Burns, who says:

> *I spent the first several years of my career doing full-time brain research on brain serotonin metabolism, but I never saw any convincing evidence that any psychiatric disorder, including depression, results from a deficiency of brain serotonin. In fact, we cannot measure brain serotonin levels in living human beings so there is no way to test this theory. Some neuroscientists would question whether this theory is even viable, since the brain does not function in this way, like a hydraulic system.*
>
> ~David Burns, 2006, author of *When Panic Attacks: The New Drug-Free Anxiety Therapy that can Change Your Life*

So, if there's no imbalance for the drugs to correct, what exactly do they do to the brain? Whitaker's book had about ten years of extra information that hadn't been available for Glenmullen at the time he wrote his book. I read on with both curiosity and apprehension—for myself and for my daughter, hoping to unravel the mystery that had played such a central role in my life.

I was confused and upset as I continued reading. Steve Hyman, the director of the National Institute of Mental Health (NIMH) from 1996 to 2001, talked about the drugs causing disruptions in the neurotransmitters, not fixing them. Because the brain wants to maintain its normal functioning, it compensates by either flooding the synapses with more of the chemical or by decreasing both the chemical and the density of the receptors for the neurotransmitter. The brain can compensate for a while, but after a time, the system breaks down, and the brain functions abnormally.[58]

Wow. So, the drugs themselves cause the chemical imbalances? How could that be? And what happens to people who take the drugs for a long time? The information was astounding. Now the idea of Prozac poop-out, where you need to increase your dose every so often to get the same result, made sense. It also made sense why it had taken me so long to get off of Elavil. I remembered that every time I tapered off the drug, within a few days my headache came raging back. I realized that I had to cut back even more gradually, nearly shaving pieces off the pill to slow my tapering.

When I read about how the drugs changed the brain, I remembered how both Dr. Sherman and Dr. Phillips, the doctor that I saw at Hopkins, had told me that antidepressants can sometimes *reveal* a bipolar condition that was already there—by flipping people into mania and moving them from depression to bipolar disorder. That explanation made no sense to me. Neither doctor disclosed the real truth: that the drugs themselves change the functioning of the brain; such a change is considered a medically induced illness or iatrogenesis (a disorder induced or created by physician or by medication). That information was in the literature, beginning in a 1956 paper by George Crane, who talked about antidepressant-induced mania. Researchers at Yale studied patients diagnosed with anxiety and depression between 1997 to 2001 and discovered that "those treated with antidepressants converted to bipolar disorder at the rate of 7.7% per year." And Fred Goodwin warned in a 2005 interview that "If you create iatragenically bipolar patient, that patient is likely to have recurrences of bipolar illness even if the offending antidepressant is discontinued."[59]

As I read the chapter on bipolar disorder, I felt like I'd escaped some awful tragedy that I had no idea existed—that my "expansive mood" or "mild, atypical hypomania" could have indeed been brought on by antidepressants, and worse yet, I could have developed an actual bipolar disorder due to the medications.

I had to keep reading to see if I was on the right track, because, obviously, after several years of being antidepressant-free, I was completely stable and had no symptoms of either depression or bipolar disorder. I hoped that Eileen would be as lucky, especially if she got off the Wellbutrin after she began to feel better. Whitaker's book presented a more complex picture than I had ever imagined. I was eager to know more.

Chapter 23: Hidden in Plain Sight

My outcome from discontinuing all psychiatric medications has been excellent—a stable mood for twenty years and a good supply of coping mechanisms to use when life gets rocky. Yet Dr. Sherman had warned me that I would relapse and become even more depressed.

Despite the good results I've experienced, I recognize that my own life story isn't enough to show that someone could remain in a stable mood without drugs. What did the research show about long-term use of psychiatric drugs? What were the outcomes for people who stayed on meds versus those who discontinued them?

NIMH looked back at surveys and studies from the 1930s and '40s up to the '70s and considered incidents of depression, rates of disability, use of medication, and recovery. They concluded that because "spontaneous recovery rates were so high, exceeding 50% within a few months, that it was difficult to judge the efficacy of a drug, a treatment (electroshock) or psychotherapy in depressed patients...and depression will run its course and terminate with virtually complete recovery without specific intervention."

Dr. Sherman had told me once or twice, "No one stays depressed forever," but I'm fairly certain that he wasn't talking about recovery without chemical intervention.[60]

As I read all of this, I felt angry and betrayed. Why had my doctors and therapists—all of them—insisted that I just needed to find the right medication? Why didn't anyone ever reassure me that I could work through things with therapy alone? But most of all, why didn't anyone warn me that I could actually get *worse* with medication? Most of the research indicated that the old treatments for depression—tricyclic antidepressants—were no better than the newer treatments—SSRIs. As early as the 1960s and '70s, doctors in Europe began warning that depression could actually be exacerbated with the use of drugs and that episodes of depression could become more frequent. Doctors found that people who took antidepressants had a more chronic form of the condition and that if they stopped taking the drugs they got much worse. NIMH concluded that patients treated with cognitive therapy alone did much better in the long run than patients taking antidepressants.[61] At the very least, Dr. Farmington and Dr. Sherman should have been aware of the ongoing debates about medication.

The information that angered me the most came from an Italian doctor's research. In 1994 (right after my final episode of depression began) Giovanni Fava of the University of Bologna wrote an editorial in *Psychotherapy and Psychosomatics* and expressed his concerns politely, yet forcefully:

> *I wonder if the time has come for debating and initiating research into the likelihood that psychotropic drugs actually worsen, at least in some cases, the progression of the illness which they are supposed to treat.... Use of antidepressants may propel the illness to a more malignant and treatment unresponsive course.*[62]

Here's what came through loud and clear for me, despite some of the unfamiliar medical language: antidepressants were pretty much no better than placebos and using antidepressants might actually make depression worse. Could that be one of the reasons why my depression had hung on for so long? The drugs weren't fixing the brain, they were contributing to the problem.[63] I remember reading this particular information and saying over and over *Thank God, I'm all right. Thank God, I got off the drugs.*

And what about the side effects, especially from the newest

antidepressants? My doctors and therapists had largely brushed off my questions, assuring me that the most severe effects happen to very few people. But I had experienced numerous side effects from many of the drugs I took, beginning with Elavil which severely impaired my ability to have any orgasms until I was able to cut way back on the dosage, below what is considered therapeutic for depression or pain management. This situation not only saddened and frustrated me, but it led to some ugly scenes between my ex and myself. Then there was the severe agitation I felt while I took Effexor, followed by the hand tremors, weight gain, fatigue, and brain fog I experienced with Depakote.

But worst of all, I kept telling the doctors that I couldn't feel—that it was as if I were living in a glass box where I could see life, but I couldn't feel it. That condition has a name as well—psychic numbing or emotional blunting—probably brought about by the dangerous combination of opioids, Valium, and Elavil. That lack of being able to feel anything is what consumed me with suicidal thoughts on a regular basis.[64] I see suicidal thinking as a side-effect now that, at the very least, was compounded by the effects of the drugs I took. For a more metaphysical explanation, Kelly Brogan, a psychiatrist who specializes in holistic treatments for depression, had this this to say about suicidal thoughts:

> *Rather, I perceive that something in them [patients] needs to die in order for them to be reborn and that this [feeling about suicide] is their raising of the white flag. This surrender is the end of the end and the beginning of the beginning, if we only let the pain come up, come out, and leave. And it does, it moves. It changes. And often, what comes in its wake is exactly the kind of shift that could never have been prescribed, taught, or suggested. It's deep spiritual growth.... Transformation requires the death of an old self. Of old beliefs. Old forms of security and identity. Transformation is disorienting and even terrifying.*[65]

I've recently begun to see the term *treatment-resistant depression* when doctors refer to people who don't respond to psychiatric drugs. But here's my bias, based on my experience and my mother's. Why don't doctors question *the treatment itself* instead of giving people more and more drugs? In the past several years, doctors have discovered that people taking antidepressants may improve initially, only to fall into a state of chronic depression. Researchers think that for some people, the very drugs used to treat depression may induce more depression, rather than relieve it. And even worse, sometimes the depressed state becomes irreversible.[66] I can't think of a crueler irony. And while this information is in the scientific literature, I have yet to see it covered in the mainstream media that most people read.

I kept reading, ever grateful that I had stopped taking antidepressants and Valium, and I was more determined than ever to help my daughter get off of her medications. She'd been in therapy for several months and was doing very well with resolving her problems and gaining new insights. At some point in her recovery, I began sharing my concerns about her taking Wellbutrin indefinitely, something her psychiatrist was recommending. I found a way to support Eileen's progress and to discuss some of the concerns I had after reading *Anatomy of an Epidemic*.

Thankfully, Eileen didn't feel the need to stay on medication, but when she broached the subject with her doctor, the doctor discouraged her. I suggested, "Why not ask her to put you on a lower dose for maintenance and see how you do?" Eileen's doctor agreed. She stayed on a lower dose for another month or so and then asked for a further reduction, finally deciding to taper off the meds slowly during the next couple of months—over her doctor's objections.

Perhaps because Eileen had observed my ability to maintain a balanced mood without drugs, she felt confident enough to try the same route. Happily, she has been able to use the tools she honed during therapy and is still managing life's ups and downs quite well.

I thought back to the last time that I'd seen Dr. Sherman. I remembered his slumped posture and what I had always considered his relaxed demeanor. The puzzle pieces fell into place for me when I realized that he was probably so calm because of emotional blunting, due to taking Prozac and Xanax, not because of his inherent nature. He had told me previously that he was taking some psych meds, but never specified which ones. And because he was willing to settle for living with drugs "that had completely destroyed [his] libido," he deemed it acceptable for his patients to make similar bargains—settling for the "security" of life book-ended with numerous side effects from psych drugs versus developing inner resources to manage life's challenges and uncertainty.

And while I'm not angry with him for his insistence that I stay on maintenance medications, I wonder: What did he know about all of the studies that I'd discovered? So many of them were released during the course of my treatment. Does he know now? I'm glad that I walked away from him that day and took the risk that I could handle anything that life threw in front of me. Without medication.

Chapter 24: Answers Regarding Recovery—It's Complicated

> *".... have patience with everything unresolved in your heart and to try to love the questions themselves."*
> ~Rainer Marie Rilke, Letters to a Young Poet

I spent a lot of time reflecting on my journey through the medical system while struggling to find healing for emotional distress. The best explanation I can offer for the reason we experience periods of darkness is this: I believe that life gives you circumstances that are challenging so that you can work out your soul's purpose and claim the life that you were meant to have. Thomas Moore, in *Care of the Soul*, explains the gifts of depression this way: "In...darkness there is to be found a precious brilliance, our essential nature, distilled by depression as perhaps the greatest gift of melancholy."

The experience of depression offered me one of life's greatest gifts: claiming my voice. Working with professionals who didn't help me or who seemed contemptuous forced me to advocate for myself and demand better care. I grew stronger with each new challenge so that I could finally stand up to my husband and leave an abusive marriage.

Understanding the mind-body connection was another important facet of my recovery. My mother's experience with severe dental pain that masked her depression had launched my journey toward understanding that connection. Fully incorporating that knowledge evolved incrementally over my lifetime, and I was beginning to put all of the pieces together in my early forties when I experienced the migraine. But, sadly, no doctor took me seriously enough to help me figure out the source of the pain.

Many doctors relegate such pain to the margins and use the dismissive term *psychosomatic illness*. That way, doctors can nod their collective heads at a patient, give her an antidepressant and an anti-anxiety drug, and tell her to come back in six months. Our Western medical model functions as if there is an impenetrable wall between the brain and the rest of the body. In reality, we are one complex, interconnected system that operates with the goal of steering us toward wholeness.

And, thankfully, some doctors recognize the power of the mind-body connection. Michael Greenwood and Peter Nunn, doctors specializing in the treatment of chronic pain, believe "all diseases have a physical, mental, emotional, spiritual, and environmental aspect. And to begin to see the connection between mind and body is to begin to see the connection between all aspects of ourselves, and of ourselves to the universe."

And as Greenwood and Nunn point out in *Paradox and Healing*, bodily pain is sometimes the only way that the psyche can focus our attention on an untenable situation. I believe that my experience with the mysterious migraine and nearly intractable depression were the tools that my psyche used to signal me that I needed to leave my husband—a man who had verbally and emotionally abused me throughout the entire time I was with him. But I didn't understand that Randy and I were dancing together as part of a system, and I had no idea how I'd gotten into such a marriage.

About a year or so after I'd gotten divorced, I heard Dr. Susan Weitzman on a radio show talking about her new book called *Not to People Like Us: Hidden Abuse in Upscale Marriages*. I think it was the first time I'd ever heard anyone talk about patterns of abuse and how systematically an abuser takes control of his partner and breaks her down. I remember feeling sick to discover that just like behavior patterns in alcoholic families and marriages, there were behavior patterns in abusive relationships. As I read through the questions that Dr. Weitzman included on her website to help you determine if you were being abused, I felt sick to my stomach at all the signs I could say yes to:

> Trying to predict your spouse's mood and anticipate behavior, trying to please your mate so he won't become angry, your mate makes impossible demands about your appearance or your weight, humiliates or belittles you in front of others. And subjects you to constant criticism and verbal rage attacks.

I was deeply upset. Why hadn't any of my therapists ever brought up the idea that maybe I was being abused? I'd told them all of these things—about Randy's rages, his constant demands for me to lose weight, the way I did things just to avoid confrontation. But once I'd calmed down over a few days and had a chance to think about everything, I felt comforted, in a way, that at least I wasn't alone. And that no matter what anyone might say or think, I'd been right to leave him.

I began looking for other books on verbal abuse and found one by Patricia Evans called *The Verbally Abusive Relationship*. She pointed out many things that helped me understand how I had stayed in such an awful marriage for such a long time. For one, many women who are in abusive relationships have been abused by people in their families. But no one in my family ever treated me the way that Randy did, I told myself. Until I read about "mean teasing" as a form of abuse. Evans says that abuse disguised as jokes "is not done in jest. It cuts to the quick, touches the most sensitive areas, and leaves the abuser with a look of triumph." Another puzzle piece dropped into place.

My dad had always teased me—many times until I cried. Then his smile would turn into a scowl and his cheery voice would bark, "Can't you take a joke? You know I'm teasing. You're just too sensitive." Evans calls these kinds of remarks *discounting*, a way to "deny and distort the partner's actual perceptions of abuse…one of the most insidious forms of abuse." And then I thought of all of my uncles—the ones who'd slapped me on the butt when I was a chubby teen and called me *Jell-O* for years. And the boyfriends who'd teased me and threatened to embarrass me, only to pull me into a hug and assure me that it was all a joke. All of the significant men in my life had treated me the same way as Randy, at least as far as the mean teasing went. So, yes, I was used to being abused. Mean teasing was a mask of love that I recognized. Even though it hurt.

Mean teasing taught me to believe that the problem was all mine, because I just couldn't take a joke and was too sensitive. Even though intellectually I knew that I *could* take a joke and *did* have a good sense of humor, I'd internalized that message after hearing it so many times. My siblings believed it as well, because our dad had always held to that opinion. "Too sensitive" was almost my middle name. Then when my husband repeated the same words over and over during our marriage, the message found the groove in my psyche and just continued to play.

Like many victims of verbal and emotional abuse, I was in denial because the abuse was perpetrated by a loved one. And I remember how long it took me to realize I was being abused. But as my son told me when I was tearfully apologizing to him for staying in a bad marriage for so long, "You can't see it until you see it."

One of the unexpected benefits of leaving my abusive marriage is that I no longer experience any depression. It's even hard for me to believe, especially based on my long history of repeated episodes. In addition to all that I've learned about the relative ineffectiveness of antidepressants, which led me to question the whole chemical imbalance theory, my own life experience stands in opposition to the theory. And even my stressful life experiences—going through a divorce, starting new jobs, losing both parents, moving—have not resulted in depression. So, I've had to consider other possibilities to explain my past experiences of dark moods, chronic pain, and suicidal thinking.

I don't believe that depression is a mental illness. I believe that depression results from serious life challenges such as trauma, abuse, chronic pain, and stress. Everyone I've ever known who has had an experience with depression has a very good reason for feeling that way. Bessel Van Der Kolk, psychiatrist and author of *The Body Keeps the Score*, says that "more than half the people who seek psychiatric care have been assaulted, abandoned, neglected, ...raped as children, or have witnessed violence in their families." Human beings need certain things in order to be healthy: they need safety and a place to live. They need love and attention on a consistent basis. They need food. They need to have their personal space—physical and mental—respected. When those conditions are violated, missing, or disregarded, our psyches can't function optimally. We feel out of balance and develop symptoms that mirror our inner distress.

Even in the 1950s, most psychiatrists understood that sympathy and time were the most important therapeutic tools for helping patients through severe emotional pain.[67] But our modern mindset almost worships the notion of a magic-bullet solution. Nothing is more difficult to witness than someone in distress, and our natural human instincts are to help solve the problem if we can. The causes of our feelings are especially troublesome to address because they are so often buried and hidden from our rational minds. I think that's why our society is easily persuaded that depression is an actual brain illness due to a chemical imbalance that can be solved by taking pills.

Many people believe that depression is hereditary, but I think it's much subtler than a transfer of actual genes from one generation to another. From an early age, I observed that my mother got lots of support and attention due to her depression. Because we all wanted to help Mom, she was relieved of many responsibilities that healthy wives and mothers would be obligated to take care of, such as grocery shopping, assisting in our classrooms, taking us places, and preparing holiday meals.

Years later, when I learned about the idea of a benefit or payoff for illness, I was outraged. What payoff was I getting for living with a migraine and chronic depression? In retrospect, I can see that the biggest payoff was that everyone around me lowered their expectations, and I had more space to reflect on my situation and do the spiritual work that was so helpful. I could also use my experience of depression to distance myself from Randy, avoiding intimacy. While I was very upset when Randy would say things like

"I'm not as attracted to you now that you're so puffy," my excess weight allowed me to avoid intimacy that I no longer wanted to share with him. And those refusals led to verbal abuse that exacerbated the depression and migraine, yet revealed the underlying problem at the same time.

I will admit that I have no definitive answer when people ask me how I finally got well. But I do have an answer for what helped me the most—spiritual practices and poetry. In the 1990s, doctors and therapists were all on the same page with how to heal depression—take pills and go to therapy, but the emphasis was always on finding the right pill. I think the therapy, in my case, was geared toward helping me sort out the problems in my marriage and to work on my wobbly self-esteem, which drove me to take on more and more responsibilities so that I could be recognized for my accomplishments. But I wanted an answer for the why of depression, both for myself and for my mother. I believed that getting to the why held the answer to getting well.

That *why* came to me when I first encountered a poem by Mary Oliver called "The Journey" on a David Whyte CD called *The Poetry of Self Compassion*. I remember the first time I heard the words "One day you finally knew / what you had to do" and "It was late / enough, and a wild night, / and the road full of fallen / branches and stones," and lastly, "determined to do / the only thing you could do— / determined to save / the only life you could / save." Finally, someone knew how I felt and understood what was going on inside of me. I wasn't trying to fix my chemicals, I was trying to fix my life.

"The Journey" met me where I was, and like all good poetry, the words and the images called forth what was working deep in my subconscious. I mulled the ideas over and over in my mind. What journey was I on? Why did it feel so scary and perilous? And why was it so clear to me that taking this journey was an attempt to save my life? I journaled about these things, I talked to the women in my prayer group, and I discussed them with my therapist. But I was the one who had to find the answers, and poetry gave me the clues I was searching for.

Whyte also explored the opening lines of Dante Alighieri's epic poem *The Inferno*. Again, as if speaking to me across time, Dante's words resonated with my experience: "In the middle of my life, I awoke in a dark wood." I had a felt-sense of what it's like to be lost in the woods, especially in the dark, and the terror that can grip you. What I was feeling had happened to millions of people throughout the ages. I didn't have an abnormal brain. I had profound life questions to wrestle with, just like people in fourteenth-century Florence.

I wish I could point to something concrete and specific, but I cannot explain why I haven't had any incidents of depression since 1997. It's not that I haven't had times of struggle and loss, but, somehow, I've avoided sinking into bleakness again. I use numerous self-care tools like regular acupuncture, daily meditation, journaling, and walking. I have many friends and a life that I'm happy with. I love my kids. But most of all, I have autonomy. I no longer live with someone who is constantly criticizing and undermining me. Still, if I ever again feel the weight of depression bearing down on me, I'll know that my soul is calling out because something in my psyche needs my loving attention.

My breakthrough with managing anxiety resulted from puzzling over David Whyte's description of Beowulf needing to go into the lake and slay Grendel's mother after he had already killed Grendel. Whyte framed the trial as being deeper that you could ever imagine: "It's not the thing you fear; it's the mother of the thing you fear." I began to notice that anxiety would grip me on the first day of every new semester when I had to meet my students. Like tapes on an endless loop, "They won't like me. My students will think I'm dumb" played endlessly in my head until I felt so sick I could barely walk into the classroom.

I tried countering the thoughts with reality: I got good evaluations, and my students regularly came to see me even after the semester was over. My colleagues respected me. Where did these feelings of inadequacy come from? And why had I felt like I was never good enough for as long as I could remember? My feelings were more visceral, more primal than fear related to student rejection. What was the mother of the thing I feared? I was stuck on the word *mother*. Then I remembered an incident from high school when I overheard a dark family secret. I don't remember who was talking, but the words they spoke were clearly about me: "Mark told me once that Helen had a hard time when Ann was a baby. As much as she wanted a daughter, Helen was consumed with thoughts about doing something awful to hurt Ann…like putting her in the oven or something."

Could that be true? My parents had always told me how happy they were when they brought me home, wrapped in "that little pink blanket." Later when I found Dad and spoke to him in the kitchen, he explained the story this way:

"Your mother was overwhelmed and had a bit of a postpartum depression after you were born. She hadn't had a baby in twelve years, and, of course, she wanted you. She was thrilled when you arrived, but you caused some upheaval in her life…"

I never forgot the way I learned of that sad truth. And puzzling over the incident years later, I realized I'd finally unearthed the roots of my anxiety. I'd found——almost literally——the mother of the thing I feared. The rejection that I felt was primal, pre-linguistic, and fierce.

Over the years, I've come to see anxiety in a new way—the overwhelming feelings come up because I have the psychic strength to overcome them and to finally let them go. I see them coming, like a gigantic wave in the ocean. I know it could smash me into the sand. But as the wave gets closer, I realize that I can ride it, and if I do crash, I know how to roll and curl into a ball. I'll be OK. I use positive self-talk to drive out the unreasonable thoughts and a few drops of Kava Kava or a pastille of Rescue Remedy, an herbal preparation that is used to help with tension and anxiety. People ask if those remedies work and I answer, "They work for me." Even in those situations that are difficult for me, I know that I have the tools to get through, and that my herbal remedies won't lead me down the dark road of dependence.

I've never been prone to headaches and usually only get them when I'm sick with a cold or the flu. But about once a year, the migraine will return. Because of all that I've learned about the mind-body connection, I see that as a sign that my life is out of balance. I don't always identify the cause, but I immediately begin to use more Five Flower essence and lavender essential oil—two things I never would have believed would help with a migraine. I imagine the headache as a circle that's getting progressively smaller and tell myself *You don't have to pay attention to this*. If I can't resolve the headache in a week, I call my energy healer for a session, which usually takes care of the pain in a few days. She helps me to pull apart the hidden sorrows in my spirit so that I can bring them to consciousness and get back to health.

While many people may question my decision to *never* take psychiatric drugs again, I would hope that all of us would agree that we deserve fully informed consent before taking any medication, but especially medications that can so profoundly affect our physical, emotional, and mental well-being. Informed consent would tell people about the placebo effect of antidepressants as well as warn of the potential for problems, including the possibility of inducing bipolar illness, creating a chronic state of depression, and struggling with an array of negative effects should one decide to withdraw from the drugs. Informed consent also includes a frank discussion of alternative treatments. Sadly, I've found websites and books to be far better sources than I ever found with my doctors. That situation needs to change. And we must demand it.

Chapter 25: The Answers in the Attic

Helen's Choices, 1937

Did my mother ever weigh her options?
Sometimes I look at her designs,
try to tease out the answer
to a puzzle I can never solve.

Was it the way my father's hand
secured
the small of her back
that signaled he was the one for her?

Was it plans for their life together—
safety, security—that Mark promised
as he slipped a square-cut diamond
onto her slender finger?

I can almost hear my grandmother mutter
Helen, don't put your faith in dreams
as she spies my grandfather tuck a pencil behind his ear
and head to the track again.

Did Mom's design instructor encourage her to pursue her gifts?
Helen, dream of dancing in that dress
Pointing to the canvas, prodding, suggesting—
imagine how silk flows, how velvet shimmers.

When potential collided with practical,
my mother chose Mark's hand.
When she tucked her designer dreams into brown cardboard—
was she hoping for a later rendezvous
with her other love?

As a family, we rarely talked about mental illness when I was a young girl. Nevertheless, compelled by the need to make sense of a senseless situation, I formed some idea of what was wrong with my mother. One of the places I searched for answers was in books. I remember reading *Jane Eyre* at about ten years old and being fascinated by Mr. Rochester's wife who was locked up in the attic. Though I didn't know it at the time, I think I identified her plight with that of my mother, being hidden away and guarded by her minder. My mother's illness was certainly hidden, at least in the sense that none of the adults in my life spoke of it in anything but a whisper.

I remember snippets of conversation where Dad talked about how my grandmother favored Mom's older sister and that Mom never felt like she got as much attention. Dad also alluded to my grandmother as being a controlling force in Mom's life. Though by the time I could understand their relationship dynamics a little better, it seemed to me that Grandma took over because Mom often collapsed and said she couldn't do something. Grandma encouraged Mom as far as I can remember. It was Dad who seemed perturbed with my grandmother, even though he relied on her to raise us while Mom was hospitalized. I sensed there was a rift between the two of them, but it remained politely subterranean.

Dad and Grandma also frequently spoke of Mom's artistic ability and how she had attended the College of Art, but I had no idea of the kind of talent my mother possessed. Once when I begged Mom for art lessons, she hung her head and said, "I can't draw." I never saw Mom paint or draw for fun or take an art class, though she encouraged my sister to pursue painting. And none of us ever knew that Mom did anything with her artistic ability except to work in the art department at Millbank's—an up-scale department store in Baltimore that was known for its fine merchandise. Sadly, Dad made her quit once they wed.

By the late nineties, Mom had developed terrible lateral stenosis—deterioration of the spinal column on one side—and because she had so much trouble walking, we moved her into a nursing home. One day when I was visiting Dad, he motioned for me to follow him down to the basement. "I want to give you my father's poetry, since you're the only writer in the family." I followed him down the worn steps and entered the storage space. The walls were still white, even after sixty years, but scarred with scrapes from moving bikes and hanging up tools. The pine shelves groaned and bowed with the weight of numerous, unlabeled, dusty boxes. While Dad pulled out a few cartons and rooted through them searching for the poetry, I noticed a slim art portfolio tucked between boxes. When I opened it, I discovered Mom's original, watercolor fashion designs and figure drawings from her time in art school. The paper was in perfect condition, and the colors were as rich and vibrant as the day Mom painted them. I was stunned by their beauty.

"Dad, look at these paintings."

He turned around and glanced at the designs as I displayed them. "That's just some stuff of your mother's." He turned back to the boxes. "The real treasure is in your grandfather's poetry."

"Dad, no, these are amazing." How could he blow off the talent so evident in these paintings? "Can I have them?"

"Sure, sure, take them all."

I went home and showed Randy and the kids, who were as impressed with Mom's talent as I was. When I took them to be framed a few days later, the man helping me asked, "Who did these? Some famous designer?"

"No, my mother."

"A collector would pay lots of money for them. They're in perfect condition."

I smiled. *Go, Mom.* "Well, they're not for sale. I want to have them framed and take them to my mother."

A few weeks later I picked up the framed paintings of Mom's dress designs and took them to the nursing home to surprise her. With the permission of the charge nurse, I set up the paintings in the sunroom so that she could get the full effect of seeing her collection. I went to her room, helped her to change into a pretty outfit, combed her hair, and applied her lipstick.

"You're getting me all dolled up. Is something special going on?"

"You'll see. I want you to look nice for your surprise."

I wheeled her down the hall into the dayroom and told her, "Don't look until I give you the signal." Once I had Mom in the sunroom, I positioned her wheelchair in front of the pictures. "Open your eyes."

Mom gasped and put her hands up to her mouth. I saw tears in her eyes, and she squeezed my hand. "Thank you for appreciating me."

Those simple words echo in my memory every time I think about that day. Mom's modest wish to have her art validated. Then she surprised me even more. "I always wanted to be a fashion designer."

Never in my life had she told me that. Not when her mother taught me to sew at thirteen. Not as she and my grandmother made pinch-pleated draperies, dust ruffles, and pillows, and not as she watched me make nearly all of my clothes and then start a sewing business. Mom had buried her gift so completely that she never shared her secret desire with anyone. I wish with all of my heart that I'd asked her more questions. But the only question that came to me was to ask if her instructors encouraged her.

"Oh, yes," she told me. "They all loved my work." Then she pointed to an exquisite painting of a woman wearing a sheer, peach-colored gown sitting with her back to the viewer. The woman's hands and face aren't visible. "That one's my favorite," Mom said. "I remember that one."

It may be a leap to say this, but I think the woman in the painting represents an aspect of my mother. I say this because as a poet, the characters in my poems usually reflect some aspect of myself or a quality I'm familiar with. My mother was beautiful and graceful like the woman in the painting. She had brown, marcel-waved hair and a slender figure, like the woman in the painting. And my mother had an aspect of modesty and reserve, like the woman in the painting. And, sadly, maybe she felt invisible, like the woman in the painting whose hands and face are hidden from view.

I remember hanging the paintings in my living room so that I could see them all the time. After my mother died I made greeting cards with her designs, sent them to my friends, and gave them as gifts. I placed Mom's bio on the back of the cards and expressed my wish for people to follow their dreams as a possible antidote to depression. I remember saying to myself over and over, "I'll never be like my mother," thinking that I would honor my soul's longings and refuse to be locked into a life without passion. But one day a voice inside whispered to me, *If you only write poetry in the summer when you aren't teaching, you might be just like your mother—by not expressing the gift that you hold most dear: your writing.*

With the discovery of my mother's paintings and my thoughts about the role of art in maintaining mental health, I formed a hypothesis about why my mother never recovered. Mom had a great talent that was never recognized beyond giving it lip-service, she had a strong-willed mother who was difficult to please and a controlling husband, and then she struggled to manage four small children born in a seven-year timespan. Because she didn't know what else to do, she self-medicated with alcohol, probably to mitigate some of the agitation and insomnia effects of the drugs. According to all the information I'd read, the combination of those factors contributed to depression—especially the use of drugs and alcohol, substances which work against each other in the body. But once I found my father's records, buried in my sister's attic years after both parents were dead, I knew I'd found the missing pieces of her story.

Just like all of Dad's other records, the file was labeled in his handwriting, and all of the papers were fastened inside with one of those pronged clips that you use to secure hole-punched pages. Dad had organized the papers by type, and I could quickly see that he'd saved insurance reimbursement forms, prescription records, his hand-drawn spreadsheets detailing Mom's medications, and letters he'd written to doctors and hospitals. On top of the pile there was a half-sheet of paper with the dates of Mom's ECT treatments with Dr. Perry. Directly underneath that paper were pages from a 1959 pharmacy bill sent by the hospital where Mom spent six months after Kelly was born. And under that was a letter with the answers to many of my previous questions about why my mother never got well. Her doctors loaded her up with pills from the very beginning and kept shoveling them into her for the rest of her life, despite never seeing any lasting improvement in her mood.

It took me months to process the information that I found in my father's files. At first, I was too enraged to write about it, because it seemed to me that even back then the doctors should have known that giving someone so many drugs and ECT treatments could be harmful.

I've come to believe, from all that I've read, that Mom's doctors, shaped by the prevailing attitudes of the time, worked within the confines of the predominant worldview of women in the fifties. They were supposed to be content and fulfilled in their sanctioned roles of housewife and mother. They were supposed to find joy in shiny appliances and spotless laundry. They were supposed to welcome each new baby with love and adjust to what was deemed a natural phenomenon. And if the woman in question had any problems with those expectations, then benevolent male doctors who knew scientific methods could chemically fix their problems.

I think that Mom's problem was largely driven by the gap between what she had the energy to accomplish and the harsh societal expectations of the time, coupled with her own high standards. Even now, women struggle to get appropriate help for postpartum depression. Many women continue to buy into the huge expectations for how they should feel when they have a new baby, but at least we now understand more about new mothers' struggles against the combined effects of sleep-deprivation and fluctuating hormones. Kelly Brogan, a psychiatrist practicing in New York who specializes in treating women holistically, has this to say about postpartum depression:

> *Many studies indicate that mothers who feel that they are receiving inadequate childcare support from the father or her family are more likely to be diagnosed with postpartum depression. That is, a mother's feelings of overwhelm, tiredness, and depletion are often categorized as postpartum depression. It has been hypothesized that the symptoms of postpartum depression may serve as a signal that the mother requires more support.*[68]

A mother requires more support. So simple to write; so difficult to implement. My mother was forty-five years old when she had my youngest sister. She had three other children ages seven, five, and three and a half. Because Dad was a supervisor, he worked shift work in rotations of 8:00 a.m. to 4:00 p.m., 4:00 p.m. to 12:00 a.m., and 12:00 a.m. to 8:00 a.m. I remember Mom's struggles to keep all of us quiet while Dad slept upstairs when he worked the nightshift. Like many families of the time, we had one car, which my father used to go to work. Most of the time, Mom was at home all day with us kids and had no means of transportation, so she couldn't even pile all of us in the car and go visit a friend if she needed some company.

Mom was also a devout Catholic, and the dictates of the time held that married women were to "welcome children lovingly from God." Mom always said she wanted to have lots of children. But welcoming them and managing them are two different things. My mother had a strong sense of duty and propriety, and based on what I saw of how she handled pain, I'm pretty sure that she internalized her struggles and attributed her feelings of being overwhelmed or distressed to her own failings.

I'm amazed that Mom could function at all with the drugs that she was taking. And, of course, Mom was drinking every day—a cocktail before dinner when Dad came home from work and then wine at bedtime.

For those years in the mid-1960s, I also have good memories of my mother and what our family was like. Our tree-lined neighborhood of two-story brick houses was built in the mid-1950s and was quickly populated with two-parent families like ours, where the moms stayed home with the kids and the dads went to work every day. Mom maintained an active life for herself by creating a regular routine of weekly and monthly events. Nearly every Tuesday, Mom dressed up, usually in a suit, as she and one of my aunts met in Baltimore for lunch and a lecture series at the Walter's Art Gallery. Tuesdays were my day to come home early and make sure dinner was ready for everyone at six o'clock. Mom left me instructions on the kitchen table, and I dutifully took care of the rest.

She was always reading the latest books, and when I close my eyes, I can still see the covers of *A Silent Spring, To Kill a Mockingbird,* and *The Agony and the Ecstasy* on the coffee table next to our sofa. With her voracious appetite for literature and female companionship, it's no wonder that for many years, Mom belonged to a book club and a bridge club, both of which sometimes met at our house. Mom was always a little anxious about entertaining, as she called it, and fussed over getting the food just so—usually trying a new recipe—cleaning the house, and creating a suitable flower arrangement for the table. Mom worked in her garden during the warmer months and took great pride in all of the flowers she so lovingly cared for.

I remember my parents being very affectionate with each other—Dad would often pat Mom on her bottom when he teased her or pull her close when she walked by and kiss her in front of all of us. They clearly loved each other and went away for one or two private weekends a year while Grandma came and stayed with us.

Travel—which was always exciting to me—was a source of great anxiety for my mother. I guess she was concerned about her sleep patterns as well as the change to her fairly rigid daily routine. She had a cleaning day, an ironing day, and a shopping day, and nothing dislodged her schedule. Mom set a timer for everything she had to do—when she put the clothes in the dryer, she set a timer for when to get them out. When she sat down in the afternoon to visit with a friend or talk to one of us, she set a timer for when she needed to cook dinner. I hated those timers! *Why can't she just be spontaneous?* I remember thinking. And I remember my vehement reaction every time I used a timer to remind myself of something. In retrospect, I see that Mom was coping in the only way she could by creating a structure for herself, because so much of her life felt chaotic and unpredictable.

And given that my father never mentioned my mother's drinking patterns, I can only fault the doctors for so much. Would they have continued to prescribe barbiturates, amphetamines, and Thorazine if they had known how much alcohol she consumed? I hope not. But I'm still stuck with the question of why they gave her so many medications when there was clearly knowledge of the dangers of addiction in the case of barbiturates and amphetamines, and of tardive dyskinesia (tics) in the case of Thorazine and all of the major tranquilizers or antipsychotics.[69]

After Mom entered the nursing home in the late nineties, she developed a chronic cough that worsened every time she ate; however, when doctors performed test after test, they failed to find its cause. After a while, it seemed that no one in the family, except me, was particularly disturbed by the coughing, even though Mom would practically choke after she ate a meal and turn completely red in the face. When I'd say something to Dad about getting Mom checked, he'd shrug and say, "She's been like that for years," as if that was a reason to accept her cough, which eluded diagnosis. After many discussions, despite his initial skepticism, Dad agreed to several tests for Mom. But when all of the results were inconclusive, her cough continued unabated.

I remember one day at the nursing home when I looked for Mom in the dining room, several of the residents who usually sat with her pulled my arm as I walked by, signaling me to stop. Their faces were lined with worry as they said to me in a chorus of concern I'll never forget, "We're so glad you're here. Every day after meals your mother coughs and coughs and it's getting worse. Please tell your father and get him to do something." Once more, Dad agreed to have several tests run on Mom, but we never knew what was wrong until the day Mom's throat closed up and she could no longer swallow.

She was rushed to the hospital and given a feeding tube in addition to a large number of diagnostic tests. When I walked into her room, my father was there to give me the news. He took me out into the hall and explained, "Your mother has throat cancer, and that's why she was always coughing. The cancer has spread to her stomach and lungs, and the doctors are saying there's nothing they can do at this point." Dad looked stricken. I'm sure Mom's terminal illness was an awful shock for him.

She had to be fed using a feeding tube. Within a few days, food was pooling in her stomach indicating that her organs were shutting down. We agreed to remove the feeding tube. Mom died ten days later, just after Dad had visited her one evening. She was eighty-eight years old. For Mom to have throat cancer and not be able to speak seemed the final logic for a woman who rarely got to express herself and who was quieted again and again with drugs.

I believe our bodies become ill in ways that make sense for the difficulties we experience. In my own life, incidents of stomach and pelvic pain and a migraine all corresponded to events in my life related to those parts of my body. And though I still have some occasional bodily symptoms of anxiety, I now have tools to manage how I feel. I credit two things for my ability to stay emotionally balanced since I stopped taking psychiatric drugs: I no longer live with someone who is abusing me, and I have developed a good set of tools to manage life's challenges. My daughter, Eileen, is also doing well without medications. She has a strong support network of friends, as well as a good acupuncturist, and she is willing to seek counseling for challenges where she needs more help.

I don't think that my mother's story could have ended any other way. She and Dad did the best they could, given the times they were living in. Both of them had such hopes and dreams for themselves when they were young, and, thankfully, they had about twenty good years together of marriage and raising children before Mom's chronic depression set in. As I combed through my father's meticulous records and read the numerous letters he wrote to doctors, I was grateful that I had found them, grateful to finally have more pieces to the puzzle of my mother's life. But I wanted to tell *Mom's* story. I wanted to know what *she* thought and felt about everything. And Mom's voice was totally silent.

Thankfully, in all of those boxes of memorabilia, I found love letters that Mom had written to Dad. I finally had Mom's voice. Her voice when she was young and in love. Mischievous and playful. Flirtatious and giddy with her first and only romance.

Here is an excerpt from one of Mom's 1931 letters that she wrote to Dad when he was away working as a camp counselor in southern Maryland. Mom was almost seventeen and Dad was nearly eighteen.

Dear Mark,

This is absolutely the first time I've ever answered a letter so quickly in all my life, not even to my mother. I think you ought to be grateful because just as soon as I finished my work I sat down to answer.

I'm so glad you enjoyed the chocolate cake and I hope you got enough…

My gracious, yes, I think canoes are wonderful plans for romance but I'm afraid we didn't have the right environment. Now, if there had been a beautiful big moon to adorn the sky with its bright light reflecting on the water and you and I in the canoe everything would have been wonderful. Of course, the seats would have to be closer, but nonetheless I enjoyed every tiny little second of the canoe rides and I don't want you to think I didn't. You know you asked me that four times in the letter.

…Now, I'll tell you how I enjoyed being with you again. I just can't think of anything of importance since then and the most wonderful time I

```
had with you.  Even though it did seem terribly short
I don't know of anything I would have enjoyed better.
Now, do you believe me??

     I haven't noticed a bit of change in you, you
seem to be that same sweet romantic little Mark.  Why
on earth did you ask me that?

     I know I won't stop counting the days until I
see you again.

     …Now, I just want to see if you'll answer as
promptly as I did.

     Love, Helen
```

When I close my eyes now and think about Mom, I see pictures of her with all of us kids when she came home from the hospital for her occasional Sunday visits. Pictures of Mom at the beach, and Mom dressed up and hosting a party. Her smile was brilliant. She looks relaxed and happy, leaning up against my father or snuggling with all of us on the sofa. And, now, instead of being disappointed at all the things Mom didn't do, I marvel that she kept her life going so well, given the powerful drugs she took for so many years. My mother was amazing. Telling her story is my way of reaching back in time to heal her. To help her. And to let her know that someone heard her in the darkness.

Appendix

List of Drugs for H. Dempsey 1959–1993
Thorazine and other major tranquilizers (later referred to as antipsychotics) 17 years
Trilafon (1959)
Tindal (62-63)
Thorazine (1959, 68-72, 73-77, 77-83)
Mellaril (1977-83)

Miltown (anti-anxiety) 14 years
1959-1973

Barbiturates (1959, 1962, 1964–1973) 11 years
Amytal
Nembutal
Phenobarbital
Butisol
Butabarbital
Pentobarbital

Antidepressants (MAO inhibitors and tricyclics) (1959–1970, 1977–1983) 17 years
Nardil (MAO)
Tofranil: tricyclic
Elavil: tricyclic
Aventyl: tricyclic

SSRI: Zoloft 1993-2002? Reported by my brother, do not have records to confirm

Dalmane: benzodiazepine 1977–1983
Dilantin: anti-seizure medication, given for depression when nothing is working 1977–1983

Amphetamines/and combo-drugs
Ritalin 1959
Dexamyl (Amphetamine and barbiturate) 1959, 1965–1968 5 years

Citations for Drug Information Related to Helen Dempsey

Drugs.com. Amytal Information from Drugs.com. c2000–2018. 4 July 2018. https://www.drugs.com/sfx/amytal-sodium-sideeffects.html#moreResources. Accessed 30 January 2019.

Drugs.com. Atropine Information from Drugs.com. c2000–2018. 20 July 2018. https://www.drugs.com/mtm/atropine-injection.html. Accessed 30 January 2019.

Drugs.com. Aventyl Information from Drugs.com. c2000–2018. 7 June 2018. https://www.drugs.com/sfx/aventyl-hydrochloride-sideeffects.html. Accessed 30 January 2019.

Drugs.com. Butabarbital Information from Drugs.com. c2000–2018. 13 September 2018. https://www.drugs.com/mtm/butabarbital.html#SideEffects. Accessed 30 January 2019.

Drugs.com. Butisol Information from Drugs.com. c2000–2018. 4 July 2018. https://www.drugs.com/sfx/butisol-sodium-side effects.html. Accessed 30 January 2019.

Drugs.com. Cogentin Information from Drugs.com. c2000–2018. 30 January 2019. https://www.drugs.com/mtm/cogentin.html. Accessed 30 January 2019.

Drugs.com. Dalmane Information from Drugs.com. c2000–2018. 7 June 2018. https://www.drugs.com/sfx/dalmane-side effects.html. Accessed 30 January 2019.

Drugs.com. Dilantin Information from Drugs.com. c2000–2018. 7 June 2018. https://www.drugs.com/sfx/dilantin-side effects.html. Accessed 30 January 2019.

Drugs.com. Doriden/Glutethimide Information from Drugs.com. c2000–2018. 3 October 1997. https://www.drugs.com/mmx/glutethimide.html. Accessed 30 January 2019.

Drugs.com. Elavil Information from Drugs.com. c2000–2018. 7 June 2018. https://www.drugs.com/sfx/elavil-side effects.html. Accessed 30 January 2019.

Drugs.com. MAO-Inhibitors Information from Drugs.com. c2000–2018. 8 June 2018. https://www.drugs.com/mca/monoamine-oxidase-inhibitors-maois. Accessed 26 February 2019.

Drugs.com. Mellaril Information from Drugs.com. c2000–2018. 4 July 2018. https://www.drugs.com/sfx/dilantin-side effects.html. Accessed 30 January 2019.

Drugs.com. Miltown Information from Drugs.com. c2000–2018. 31 October 2018. https://www.drugs.com/cons/miltown.html. Accessed 30 January 2019.

Drugs.com. MS-Contin Information from Drugs.com. c2000–2018. 19 June 2019. https://www.drugs.com/cons/mscontin.html. Accessed 26 August 2019.

Drugs.com. Nardil Information from Drugs.com. c2000–2018. 6 June 2018. https://www.drugs.com/sfx/nardil-side effects.html. Accessed 30 January 2019.

Drugs.com. Nembutal Information from Drugs.com. c2000–2018. 11 July 2018. https://www.drugs.com/cdi/nembutal.html. Accessed 30 January 2019.

Drugs.com. Pentobarbital Information from Drugs.com. c2000–2018. 10 March 2017. https://www.drugs.com/mtm/pentobarbital-injection.html. Accessed 30 January 2019.

Drugs.com. Phenobarbital Information from Drugs.com. c2000–2018. 4 September 2018. https://www.drugs.com/mtm/phenobarbital.html. Accessed 30 January 2019.

Drugs.com. Prednisone Information from Drugs.com. c2000–2018. 31 October 2018. https://www.drugs.com/mtm/prednisone.html. Accessed 16 February 2019.

Drugs.com. Ritalin Information from Drugs.com. c2000–2018. 6 June 2018. https://www.drugs.com/sfx/ritalin-side effects.html. Accessed 30 January 2019.

Drugs.com. Sparine Information from Drugs.com. c2000–2018. https://www.drugs.com/sfx/sparine-side effects.html. Accessed 30 January 2019.

Drugs.com. Thorazine Information from Drugs.com. c2000–2018. 19 June 2018. https://www.drugs.com/sfx/thorazine-side effects.html. Accessed 30 January 2019.

Drugs.com. Tofranil Information from Drugs.com. c2000–2018. 6 June 2018. https://www.drugs.com/sfx/tofranil-side effects.html. Accessed 30 January 2019.

Drugs.com. Trilafon Information from Drugs.com. c2000–2018. 26 September 2018. https://www.drugs.com/mtm/trilafon.html. Accessed 30 January 2019.

Drugs.com. Zoloft Information from Drugs.com. c2000–2018. 7 June 2018. https://www.drugs.com/sfx/zoloft-side effects.html. Accessed 30 January 2019.

"Tindal Tablet - Uses, Side effects, Reviews, and Precautions - Schering - TabletWise - USA" Tabletwise.com. N.p., n.d. https://www.tabletwise.com/us/tindal-tablet. Accessed 25 January 2019.

Ann's Medications 1993–2007
Benzodiazepines and Anti-anxiety drugs
Ativan 1995, 1996
Valium, 1993–1999, 2001, 2004–2007 *(from 2001 until 2007, I'm pretty sure that I used Valium on a PRN basis.)*
Buspar, 1994

Antidepressants (16 years)
Elavil, 1993–2008 *(It took me many years to finally get off of Elavil due to rebound headaches every time I cut the dose to very low levels.)* The antidepressants below were always combined with Elavil which was originally given for headache pain.
Paxil, 1994
Nortriptyline, 1994
Zoloft, 1994
Effexor, 1994, 1995
Serzone, 1995
Wellbutrin, 1995–1996, 1999–2002

Mood regulators (7 years)
Lithium, 1994-1995
Depakote, 1995–1998
Topamax 1999–2002

Opioids (5 years)
MS-Contin, 1996
OxyContin, 1997–1998
Methadone, 1999–2000
Demerol, 1999, 2000 ((used on a PRN basis, injectable)
Percocet, 2007 (for some injury, not headache)

Beta Blockers
Lopressor, 1996

Headache Drugs
DHE-45, 1996, 1998, 1999 (injectable)
Migranol Nasal Spray, 1995–2000
Imitrex, 1995–1997

Antihistamine
Vistaril, 1997 (used to treat anxiety)

Diuretic
Bumex, 1997–1999

Steroids
Prednisone, 1996–1999 (used to reduce inflammation when headache pain escalated; oral when at home, IV when hospitalized 5 times for migraine treatment)

NSAID (used for arthritis)
Indocin, 2000–2001
Naproxen, 2001, 2002, 2008, 2009
Vioxx, 2004
Aleve, 2005–2006
Celebrex, 2007

Muscle Relaxant (I must have had an injury, not for headache or depression)
Flexeril, 2007

Organizations to Help with Psychiatric Drug Withdrawal Process
Author's note: For a variety of reasons, most physicians, nurse practitioners, and psychiatrists are poorly educated in the best ways to help people discontinue psychiatric drugs. The following organizations provide written information, suggested tapering schedules, and support groups to help people who want to discontinue their drugs.

Easing Anxiety https://www.easinganxiety.com
This website is devoted to educating people about anxiety issues and providing help for those who wish to withdraw from antianxiety drugs. They provide a link to The Ashton Manual, written by Dr. Heather Ashton, which is a complete guide to benzodiazepine drugs and suggested withdrawal processes. https://www.benzoinfo.com/wp-content/uploads/2020/08/Ashton-Manual.pdf

Harm Reduction Guide to Coming Off Psychiatric Drugs https://www.mentalhealthforum.net/resources/ComingOffPsychDrugsHarmReductGuide.pdf
This guide, published by The Icarus Project and The Freedom Center, recognizes that everyone is in a different space regarding psychiatric drugs. Their harm reduction approach educates people on the pros and cons of psychiatric drugs and then provides resources for people who decide to discontinue their drugs.

Inner Compass Initiative's Withdrawal Project https://withdrawal.theinnercompass.org
Laura Delano, a psychiatric survivor, founded the Inner Compass Initiative as a resource for people who want to be educated about all of the effects of psychiatric drugs so that they can make informed decisions about their treatment. The Withdrawal Project provides information on psychiatric drugs and many helpful resources for people who choose to discontinue their drugs.

Mad in America https://www.madinamerica.com
This website, founded by award-winning science writer Robert Whitaker, features personal stories, current research, and continuing education around mental health issues. Resources for psychiatric drug information, withdrawal, providers, and alternative treatments are also provided.

Medicating Normal https://medicatingnormal.com
The Medicating Normal Team produced a feature film documentary featuring people who struggled with the effects of overmedication and attempted to discontinue their psychiatric drugs. Psychiatrists, counselors, and pharmacists are also interviewed and provide more context for the survivors' stories. Resources to help with the withdrawal process are available on the website.

Surviving Antidepressants https://www.survivingantidepressants.org
Adele Framer founded this organization after she struggled to wean herself off of antidepressants and found no real help, even after visiting fifty psychiatrists. She did her own research using medical journals and FDA recommendations and then founded Surviving Antidepressants, a peer education and support website, in 2011.

Notes

Ch. 2 : Reflections

[1] Rasmussen, Nicholas. "America's First Amphetamine Epidemic: 1929–1970." *American Journal of Public Health.* June 2008, vol. 98, no.6, pp. 974–985. http://whale.to/a/rasmussen.html

[2] Silverman, Harold, MD. (ed). *The Pill Book: The Illustrated Guide to the Most-Prescribed Drugs in the United States.* New York: Bantam Books, 1998. Pg. 869–873 (Nardil), 1125–1132 (Tofranil).

[3] Drugs.com. Trilafon Information from Drugs.com. c2000–2018. Updated 26 September 2018. Accessed 30 January 2019 https://www.drugs.com/mtm/trilafon.html

[4] Munoz, F.L., Ucha-Udabe, R. and Alamo, C. "The History of Barbiturates a Century After Their Clinical Introduction." Neuropsychiatric Disease and Treatment. December 2005. 1(4): 329–343. www.ncbi.nlm.nih.gov/pmc/articles/PMC2424120/

[5] Rasmussen, Nicholas. "America's First Amphetamine Epidemic: 1929–1970." American Journal of Public Health. June 2008, vol. 98, no.6, pp. 974–985. http://whale.to/a/rasmussen.html

Ch. 3: Just Like Your Mother

[6] Drugs.com. Nembutal Information from Drugs.com. c2000–2018. Updated 11 July 2018. Accessed 30 January 2019 https://www.drugs.com/cdi/nembutal.html

"Drugs That Can Cause Depression, Agitation, and Suicidality" Retrieved from Rxisk, Making Medicines Safer for All of Us. Website https://rxisk.org/drugs-that-can-cause-depression-agitation-suicidality/. November 2, 2020.

Ch. 4: More is Better, But No One Mentioned the Side Effects

[7] Drugs.com. Butisol Information from Drugs.com. c2000–2018. Updated 4 July 2018. Accessed 30 January 2019. https://www.drugs.com/sfx/butisol-sodium-side-effects.html

Drugs.com. Doriden/Glutethimide Information from Drugs.com. c2000–2018. Updated 3 October 1997. Accessed 30 January 2019. https://www.drugs.com/mmx/glutethimide.html

Drugs.com. Miltown Information from Drugs.com. c2000–2018. Updated 31 October 2018. Accessed 30 January 2019. https://www.drugs.com/cons/miltown.html

Drugs.com. Tofranil Information from Drugs.com. c2000–2018. Updated 6 June 2018. Accessed 30 January 2019. https://www.drugs.com/sfx/tofranil-side-effects.html

"Tindal Tablet - Uses, Side-effects, Reviews, and Precautions - Schering - TabletWise - USA" Tabletwise.com. N.p., n.d. Web. 25 Jan. 2019.

Drugs listed in my father's records
1960–61: Tofranil & Miltown
1962: Tofranil, Tindal, NaButisol (pink and green), Doriden

[8] "Battle Against Drugs Turns to Barbiturates." Article. U. S. News & World Report. 23 April 1973. 59–60. Print.

[9] Ibid.

Ch. 6: Looking for the Why

[10] Rasmussen, Nicholas. "America's First Amphetamine Epidemic: 1929–1970." American Journal of Public Health. June 2008, vol. 98, no.6, pp. 974–985. http://whale.to/a/rasmussen.html

Drugs.com. Aventyl Information from Drugs.com. c2000–2018. Updated 7 June 2018. Accessed 30 January 2019. https://www.drugs.com/sfx/aventyl-hydrochloride-side-effects.html

Drugs.com. Pentobarbital Information from Drugs.com. c2000–2018. Updated 10 March 2017. Accessed 30 January 2019. https://www.drugs.com/mtm/pentobarbital-injection.html

https://en.wikipedia.org/wiki/Dexamyl

https://www.alternet.org/2016/10/when-meth-medicine-big-pharma-amphetamine-ads/

[11] Herzberg, David. *Happy Pills in America: From Miltown to Prozac.* Baltimore: The Johns Hopkins University Press. 2009. Print. P. 76

Ch. 7: The Long Way Around

[12] Moore, Thomas. *Care of the Soul: A Guide for Cultivating Depth and Sacredness in Everyday Life.* New York: Harper Collins, 1992. Print. Pg. 137.

[13] Greenwood, Michael, MD, Nunn, Peter, MD. *Paradox and Healing: Medicine, Mythology, and Transformation.* Victoria: Paradox Publishers. 1992. Print. Pg. 23.

[14] Hickey, Philip. Mad in America. "Antidepressant Induced Mania." 11 January 2015. Web. https://www.madinamerica.com/2015/01/antidepressant-induced-mania/

Ch. 9: If It's Not Working, Do More of It

[15] Abse, D.W., MD and J.A. Ewing, MD. "Transference and Countertransference in Somatic Therapies." The Journal of Nervous and Mental Disease 123, no. 1(1956): 32–40. https://journals.lww.com/jonmd/Citation/1956/01000/Transference_and_Counter_Transference_in_Somatic.5.aspx

[16] Herzberg, David. *Happy Pills in America: From Miltown to Prozac.* Baltimore: The Johns Hopkins University Press. 2009. Pg. 91–92.

[17] Northrup, Bowen. "Shock Treatment Remains Controversial, Though Horror of the Past is Obsolete." Wall Street Journal. 11 August 1986. Print.

[18] Abse, D.W., MD and J.A. Ewing, MD. "Transference and Countertransference in Somatic Therapies." The Journal of Nervous and Mental Disease 123, no. 1(1956): 32–40. https://journals.lww.com/jonmd/Citation/1956/01000/Transference_and_Counter_Transference_in_Somatic.5.aspx

[19] Ibid.

[20] Ibid.

[21] Burstow, Bonnie. "Electroshock as a Form of Violence Against Women." Violence Against Women. April 2006: 12(4), 372–392. http://psychrights.org/Research/Digest/Electroshock/2006Burstow-ElectroshockAsViolenceAgainst%20Women.pdf

[22] Breggin, Peter R. "The FDA Should Test the Safety of ECT Machines." International Journal of Risk and Safety in Medicine. 2010: 22, 89–92. www.ectresources.org/ECT Science/Breggin_2010_ECT_AAA_Overview_written_to_FDA_Brain_Damage_Memor y_Loss_pdf

[23] Tone, Andrea. *The Age of Anxiety.* New York: Basic Books, A Member of Perseus Books Group. 2009. Pg. 159.

[24] Herzberg, David. *Happy Pills in America: From Miltown to Prozac.* Baltimore: The Johns Hopkins University Press. 2009. Pg. 73.

[25] Northrup, Bowen. "Shock Treatment Remains Controversial, Though Horror Image of Past is Obsolete." Wall Street Journal. 11 August 1986. Print.

Ch. 11 ECT: The Backstory

[26] Burstow, Bonnie. "Electroshock as a Form of Violence Against Women." Violence Against Women. April 2006: 12(4), 372–392. Web.

[27] Breggin, Peter, R. "The FDA Should Test the Safety of ECT Machines." International Journal of Risk and Safety in Medicine. 2010: 22, 89–92. Web.

[28] Ibid. Burstow.

[29] Waikar, Arpana et al. "ECT Without Anesthesia is Unethical." Issues in Medical Ethics. April–June 2003: XI (2). Web.

Ch. 12 Down the Rabbit Hole

[30] Quinones, Sam. *Dreamland: A True Tale of America's Opiate Epidemic.* New York: Bloomsbury Press. 2015. Pgs. 124–127.

Drugs.com. MS-Contin Information from Drugs.com. c2000–2018. Updated 13 June 2019. Accessed 02 November 2020 https://www.drugs.com/ms_contin.html#moreResources

[31] Drugs.com. OxyContin Information from Drugs.com. c2000–2018. Updated 4 November 2019. Accessed 02 November 2020. https://www.drugs.com/sfx/oxycontin-side-effects.html

Ch. 13: Treatment Resistant Patient

[32] Silverman, Harold, MD. (ed). *The Pill Book: The Illustrated Guide to the Most-Prescribed Drugs in the United States.* New York: Bantam Books, 1998. Pgs. 862–863.

[33] Greenwood, Michael, MD, Nunn, Peter, MD. *Paradox and Healing: Medicine, Mythology, and Transformation.* Victoria: Paradox Publishers. 1992. Pgs. 23 & 29.

[34] El-Mallakh, R., Gao, Y. & Roberts, J. "Tardive Dysphoria: The Role of Long Term Antidepressant Use in Inducing Chronic Depression." Medical Hypotheses. 12 January 2011: 76, 769–773. Web. Pg. 771.

Fava, G. & Belaise, C. "Discontinuing Antidepressant Drugs: Lesson from a Failed Trail and Extensive Clinical Experience." Psychotherapy and Psychosomatics. vol. 87, no.5, pp. 257–267. September 2018. DOI: 10.1159/000492693.

Ch. 14: A Therapeutic Environment

[35] Silverman, Harold, MD. (ed). *The Pill Book: The Illustrated Guide to the Most-Prescribed Drugs in the United States.* New York: Bantam Books, 1998. Pgs. 255–256.

Drugs.com [Internet]. Prednisone Information from Drugs.com; c1996–2018 [Updated: 13 February 2018, Cited: 19 June 2018]. Available from: https://www.drugs.com/prednisone.html

Ch. 18: Why Didn't My Doctors Warn Me?

[36] National Institute on Drug Abuse. National Institute on Drug Abuse: Advancing Addiction Science. "Opioids and Chronic Pain: A Gap in Our Knowledge." 25 September 2014.

[37] Robert, Teri. "Medication-Overuse Headache." Very Well Health. https://www.verywellhealth.com/medications-overuse-rebound-headaches-1719183. July 10, 2019.

Kristofferson, E.S. and Lundqvist, C. "Medication-overuse headache: a review." Journal of Pain Research. 2014. 7:367–378. Doi: 10.2147/JPR.S46071. https://www.ncbi.nim.nimh.gov/pmc/articles/PMC4110872/

38 Westergaard, M.L. et al. "Medication-overuse Headache: A Perspective Review." Therapeutic Advances in Drug Safety. 2016 August. Vol. 7(4), 147–158. doi: 10.1177/2042098616653390

39 Ibid. Robert.

40 Ibid. Robert.
41 Payte, J. Thomas. "A Brief History of Methadone in the Treatment of Opioid Dependence: A Personal Perspective." Journal of Psychoactive Drugs. 1991. vol. 23, no. 2, pp. 103–107 doi: 10.1080/02791072.1991.10472226

Quinones, Sam. *Dreamland: A True Tale of America's Opiate Epidemic.* New York: Bloomsbury Press. 2015. Pg. 63.

42 "Benzodiazepines and Opioids." National Institutes of Health, U.S. Department of Health and Human Services, 16 Jan. 2022, https://nida.nih.gov/drug-topics/opioids/benzodiazepines-opioids

Silverman, Harold, MD. (ed). *The Pill Book: The Illustrated Guide to the Most-Prescribed Drugs in the United States.* New York: Bantam Books, 1998. Pgs. 300, 859, 861.

43 Quinones, Sam. *Dreamland: A True Tale of America's Opiate Epidemic.* New York: Bloomsbury Press. 2015. Pg.124.

Wikipedia contributors. "Oxycodone." Wikipedia, The Free Encyclopedia. Wikipedia, The Free Encyclopedia, 20 Aug. 2019. https://en.wikipedia.org/w/index.php?title=Oxycodone&oldid=911703226

44 United States Food and Drug Administration. "Women and Pain Factsheet." 2019. PDF.

45 *Dorland's Medical Dictionary for Consumers 2007*: polypharmacy

46 Kukreja, S. et al. "Polypharmacy in Review." Mens Sana Monographs. 2013 January–December. vol. 11, no. 1, Pgs. 82–99. www.ncbi.nlm.nih.gov/pmc/articles/PMC3653237/

Ch. 19: Paradigm Shift

[47] Glenmullen, Joseph, MD *Prozac Backlash: Overcoming the Dangers of Prozac, Zoloft, Paxil and Other Antidepressants with Safe, Effective Alternatives*. New York: Simon and Schuster, 2000. Pg. 50.

[48] Ibid. Pg. 21.

[49] Ibid. Pg. 51.

[50] Whitaker, Robert. *Anatomy of an Epidemic: Magic Bullets, Psychiatric Drugs, and the Astonishing Rise of Mental Illness in America*. New York: Broadway Paperback, 2010. Print. Pg. 51.

Ch. 20: What Could a Patient Possibly Understand About Clinical Trials?

[51] Glenmullen, Joseph, MD *Prozac Backlash: Overcoming the Dangers of Prozac, Zoloft, Paxil and Other Antidepressants with Safe, Effective Alternatives*. New York: Simon and Schuster, 2000. Pgs. 166-167.

[52] Ibid. Pg. 167.

[53] Ibid. Pg. 181.

Ch. 21: You Have a Damaged Brain

[54] Simons, Peter. Mad in America. "New Study Examines Users Experience of Discontinuing Psychiatric Medications." 26 July 2017. Web. https://www.madinamerica.com/2017/07/new-study-examines-user-experience-discontinuing-psychiatric-medications/

[55] Ibid. Glenmullen. Pgs. 166-167.

Ch. 22 The Book of Revelation

[56] Whitaker, Robert. *Anatomy of an Epidemic: Magic Bullets, Psychiatric Drugs, and the Astonishing Rise of Mental Illness in America.* New York: Broadway Paperback, 2010. Print. Pg. 53.

[57] Ibid. Pg. 68.

[58] Ibid. Pg. 83.

[59] Ibid. Pg. 181.

Ch. 23: Hidden in Plain Sight

[60] Whitaker, Robert. *Anatomy of an Epidemic: Magic Bullets, Psychiatric Drugs, and the Astonishing Rise of Mental Illness in America.* New York: Broadway Paperback, 2010. Print. Pg. 153.

[61] Ibid. Pg. 158.

[62] Ibid. Pg. 159.

[63] Ibid. Pg. 160.

[64] Breggin, Peter R. & Cohen, David. Your Drug May Be Your Problem: How and Why to Stop Taking Psychiatric Medications. Philadelphia: DaCapo Press. 1999. Print. Pgs. 72–73

[65] Brogan, Kelly. Kelly Brogan MD. *Own Your Body. Free Your Mind.* "How to Help Someone Who Is Suicidal." https://kellybroganmd.com/how-to-help-someone-who-is-suicidal/

[66] El-Mallakh, R., Gao, Y. & Roberts, J. "Tardive Dysphoria: The Role of Long Term Antidepressant Use in Inducing Chronic Depression." Medical Hypotheses. 12 January 2011: 76, 769–773.

https://www.madinamerica.com/wpcontent/uploads/2011/11/tardivedysphoriadarticle.pdf

Ch. 24 Answers Regarding Recovery: It's Complicated

[67] Rasmussen, Nicholas. "America's First Amphetamine Epidemic: 1929–1970." American Journal of Public Health. June 2008, vol. 98, no.6, Pgs. 974–985. http://whale.to/a/rasmussen.html

Ch. 25 The Answers in the Attic

[68] Brogan, Kelly. Kelly Brogan MD. *Own Your Body. Free Your Mind.* "The Many Origins of Depression. https://kellybroganmd.com/the-many-origins-of-depression.

[69] Munoz, F.L., Ucha-Udabe, R. and Alamo, C. "The History of Barbiturates a Century After Their Clinical Introduction." Neuropsychiatric Disease and Treatment. December 2005. 1(4): 329–343. www.ncbi.nlm.nih.gov/pmc/articles/PMC2424120/

References

Books

Evans, Patricia. *The Verbally Abusive Relationship: How to Recognize it and How to Respond.* Holbrook: Adams Media Corporation, 1992, 1996.

Glenmullen, Joseph, MD. *Prozac Backlash: Overcoming the Dangers of Prozac, Zoloft, Paxil and Other Antidepressants with Safe, Effective Alternatives.* New York: Simon and Schuster, 2000.

Greenwood, Michael, MD, Nunn, Peter, MD. *Paradox and Healing: Medicine, Mythology, and Transformation.* Victoria: Paradox Publishers. 1992.

Herzberg, David. *Happy Pills in America: From Miltown to Prozac.* Baltimore: The Johns Hopkins University Press. 2009.

Lynch, Terry. *Depression Delusion: The Myth of the Brain Chemical Imbalance, Vol. I.* Limerick: Mental Health Publishing. 2015. Pgs. 37, 39, 41.

Moore, Thomas. *Care of the Soul: A Guide for Cultivating Depth and Sacredness in Everyday Life.* New York: Harper Collins, 1992.

Oliver, Mary. "The Journey." *New and Selected Poems.* Boston: Beacon Press. 1992.

Quinones, Sam. *Dreamland: A True Tale of America's Opiate Epidemic.* New York: Bloomsbury Press. 2015.

Rilke, Rainer Marie. *Letters to a Young Poet.* New York: Random House. 1984.

Silverman, Harold, MD. (ed). *The Pill Book: The Illustrated Guide to the Most-Prescribed Drugs in the United States.* New York: Bantam Books, 1998.

Tone, Andrea. *The Age of Anxiety.* New York: Basic Books, A Member of Perseus Books Group. 2009.

Van Der Kolk, Bessel, MD. *The Body Keeps the Score: Brain, Mind, and Body in the Healing of Trauma.* New York: Penguin Books, 2014.

Weitzman, Susan. *Not to People Like Us: Hidden Abuse in Upscale Marriages.* New York: Basic Books. 2000. Print.

Whitaker, Robert. *Anatomy of an Epidemic: Magic Bullets, Psychiatric Drugs, and the Astonishing Rise of Mental Illness in America.* New York: Broadway Paperback, 2010. Print.

Journals and Magazines

Abse, D.W., MD and J.A. Ewing, MD. "Transference and Countertransference in Somatic Therapies." *The Journal of Nervous and Mental Disease* 123, no. 1 (1956): 32–40. https://journals.lww.com/jonmd/Citation/1956/01000/Transference_and_Counter_Transference_in_Somatic.5.aspx.

"Battle Against Drugs Turns to Barbiturates." Article. *U. S. News & World Report.* 23 April, 1973. 59–60. Print.

Breggin, Peter, R. "The FDA Should Test the Safety of ECT Machines." *International Journal of Risk and Safety in Medicine.* 2010: 22, 89–92. www.ectresources.org/ECTscience/

Breggin_2010_ECT__AAA__Overview_written_to_FDA____Brain_Damage___Memory_Loss_.pdf.

Burstow, Bonnie. "Electroshock as a Form of Violence Against Women." *Violence Against Women.* April 2006: 12(4), 372–392. http://psychrights.org/Research/Digest/Electroshock/2006Burstow-ElectroshockAsViolenceAgainst%20Women.pdf.

El-Mallakh, R., Gao, Y. & Roberts, J. "Tardive Dysphoria: The Role of Long Term Antidepressant Use in Inducing Chronic Depression." Medical Hypotheses. 12 January 2011: 76, 769–773. https://www.madinamerica.com/wp-content/uploads/2011/11/tardivedysphoriadarticle.pdf.

Fava, G. & Belaise, C. "Discontinuing Antidepressant Drugs: Lesson from a Failed Trail and Extensive Clinical Experience." *Psychotherapy and Psychosomatics.* vol. 87, no.5, pp. 257–267, September 2018. DOI: 10.1159/000492693.

Kristofferson, E.S. and Lundqvist, C. "Medication-overuse headache: a review." *Journal of Pain Research.* 2014. 7:367–378. Doi: 10.2147/JPR.S46071. https://www.ncbi.nim.nimh.gov/pmc/articles/PMC4110872/.

Kukreja, S. et al. "Polypharmacy in Review." *Mens Sana Monographs.* 2013 January-December. vol. 11, no. 1, pp. 82–99. www.ncbi.nlm.nih.gov/pmc/articles/PMC3653237/.

Mao, Jianren. "Opioid-induced abnormal pain sensitivity: implications in clinical opioid therapy." *Pain.* December 2002. vol. 10, issue 3, pp. 213–217, doi: 10.1016/S0304-3959(02)00422-0.

Munoz, F.L., Ucha-Udabe, R. and Alamo, C. "The History of Barbiturates a Century After Their Clinical Introduction." *Neuropsychiatric Disease and Treatment.* December, 2005. 1(4): 329–343. www.ncbi.nlm.nih.gov/pmc/articles/PMC2424120/.

Northrup, Bowen. "Shock Treatment Remains Controversial, Though Horror Image of Past is Obsolete." *Wall Street Journal.* 11 August 1986. Print.

Payte, J. Thomas. "A Brief History of Methadone in the Treatment of Opioid Dependence: A Personal Perspective." *Journal of Psychoactive Drugs*. 1991.vol. 23, no. 2, pp. 103–107 doi: 10.1080/02791072.1991.10472226

Rasmussen, Nicholas. "America's First Amphetamine Epidemic: 1929–1970." *American Journal of Public Health*. June 2008, vol. 98, no.6, pp. 974–985. http://whale.to/a/rasmussen.htmlWeb.

Sargant, W. "Drugs in the Treatment of Depression." *British Medical Journal* vol. 1,5221 (1961): 225-7. doi:10.1136/bmj.1.5221.225

Tompkins, D.A. & Campbell, C.M. "Opioid-Induced Hyperalgesia: Clinically Relevant or Extraneous Research Phenomenon?" *Current Pain Headache Report.* (2011) 15: 129. https://doi.org/10.1007/s11916-010-0171-1.

Waikar, Arpana et al. "ECT Without Anesthesia is Unethical." *Issues in Medical Ethics.* April-June 2003: XI (2). www.researchgate.net/publication/7433204_ECT_without_anaesthesia_is_unethical/download.

Westergaard, M.L. et al. "Medication-overuse Headache: A Perspective Review." *Therapeutic Advances in Drug Safety*. 2016 August. Vol. 7(4), 147–158. doi: 10.1177/2042098616653390

Websites

"Benzodiazepines and Opioids." *National Institutes of Health*, U.S. Department of Health and Human Services, 16 Jan. 2022, https://nida.nih.gov/drug-topics/opioids/benzodiazepines-opioids

Biancolli, Amy (2020, November 2). *Surviving Antidepressants: An Interview with Adele Framer.* [Blog post]. Retrieved from https://www.madinamerica.com/2020/11/surviving-antidepressants-adele-framer/

Brogan, Kelly. *Kelly Brogan MD: Own Your Body. Free Your Mind.* "The Many Origins of Depression." https://kellybroganmd.com/the-many-origins-of-depression/

Brogan, Kelly. *Kelly Brogan MD: Own Your Body. Free Your Mind.* "How to Help Someone Who Is Suicidal." https://kellybroganmd.com/how-to-help-someone-who-is-suicidal/

Center for Disease Control and Prevention. "Prescription Painkiller Overdoses: A Growing Epidemic, Especially Among Women." Atlanta, GA. 2013. Web. http://www.cdc.gov/vitalsigns/prescriptionpainkilleroverdoses/index.html

Dhar, Ayurdhi. (2020, November 2). Researchers: It's time to stop recommending antidepressants for depression [Blog post]. Retrieved from https://www.madinamerica.com/2020/10/researchers-suggest-antidepressants-not-used-depression/

Dorland's Medical Dictionary for Consumers. © 2007 by Saunders, an imprint of Elsevier, Inc. All rights reserved. https://medical-dictionary.thefreedictionary.com/polypharmacy

www.healthline.com/health/depression/what-are-mao-inhibitors. Accessed 26 February 2019.

Hickey, Philip. *Mad in America.* "Antidepressant Induced Mania." 11 January 2015. Web. https://www.madinamerica.com/2015/01/antidepressant-induced-mania/

Horton, Lucie *Transforming Mental Health Through Research.* "Five Ways to Treat Anxiety." 3 January 2018. Web. https://www.mqmentalhealth.org/posts/5-new-ways-to-treat-anxiety

Hyperalgesia: https://www.drugabuse.gov/about-nida/noras-blog/2014/09/opioids-chronic-pain-gap-in-our-knowledge

National Institute on Drug Abuse. *National Institute on Drug Abuse: Advancing Addiction Science.* "Opioids and Chronic Pain: A Gap in Our Knowledge." 25 September 2014.

Payte, J. Thomas. "A Brief History of Methadone in the Treatment of Opioid Dependence: A Personal Perspective." *Journal of Psychoactive Drugs.* 1991. vol. 23, no. 2, pp. 103–107 doi: 10.1080/02791072.1991.10472226

Perdue Pharma. "Oxytocin's-Contin Press Release 1996." 1996. PDF. Found in *LA Times*-Documents, Posted 5 May 2015. Accessed 24 August 2019.

Renew Medical Clinics. *Renew Medical Clinics: Methadone*, 2019. http://renewmedicalclinics.com/aboutmethadone

Robert, Teri. "Medication-Overuse Headache." *Very Well Health*. https://www.verywellhealth.com/medications-overuse-rebound-headaches-1719183. July 10, 2019.

Simons, Peter. *Mad in America*. "New Study Examines Users Experience of Discontinuing Psychiatric Medications." 26 July 2017. Web. https://www.madinamerica.com/2017/07/new-study-examines-user-experience-discontinuing-psychiatric-medications/

United States Food and Drug Administration. "Women and Pain Factsheet." 2019. PDF.

United States Food and Drug Administration. (2020 9 23). *FDA Requiring Labeling Changes for Benzodiazepines: Black Box Warning to be Updated to Include Abuse, Addiction, and Other Serious Risks* (Press Release). https://www.fda.gov/news-events/press-announcements/fda-requiring-labeling-changes-benzodiazepines

Weitzman, Susan, MD. *The Weitzman Center*. https://www.weitzmancenter.org/test/

Wikipedia contributors. "Dexamyl." *Wikipedia, The Free Encyclopedia*. Wikipedia, The Free Encyclopedia, 29 Aug. 2018. https://en.wikipedia.org/wiki/Dexamyl. Accessed 30 Jan. 2019.

Wikipedia contributors. "Methadone." *Wikipedia, The Free Encyclopedia*. Wikipedia, The Free Encyclopedia, 20 Aug. 2019. https://en.wikipedia.org/w/index.php?title=Methadone&oldid=911702963

Wikipedia contributors. "Oxycodone." *Wikipedia, The Free Encyclopedia*. Wikipedia, The Free Encyclopedia, 20 Aug. 2019. https://en.wikipedia.org/w/index.php?title=Oxycodone&oldid=911703226

CD

Whyte, David. *The Poetry of Self Compassion*. Langley: Many Rivers Press. 1992. CD

Bibliography

Books

Brennan, Barbara. *Hands of Light: A Guide to Healing Through the Human Energy Field*. New York: Bantam Books. 1988.

Websites

Bach Original Flower Remedies. A. Nelson & Company. 2019. https://www.bachremedies.com/en-us/bach-story.

Chios Energy Healing. Chios Energy Healing. 2019. https://www.chioshealing.com/HealingLevel1/ChakraSystem/chakrasystem.htm.

About the Author

Ann Bracken has published three poetry collections, *The Altar of Innocence, No Barking in the Hallways: Poems from the Classroom,* and *Once You're Inside: Poetry Exploring Incarceration.* She serves as a contributing editor for *Little Patuxent Review* and co-facilitates the Wilde Readings Poetry Series in Columbia, Maryland. She volunteers as a correspondent for the Justice Arts Coalition, exchanging letters with incarcerated people to foster their use of the arts. Her poetry, essays, and interviews have appeared in numerous anthologies and journals, her work has been featured on *Best American Poetry*, and she's been a guest on Grace Cavalieri's *The Poet and The Poem* radio show. Her advocacy work promotes using the arts to foster paradigm change in the areas of emotional wellness, education, and prison abolition.

Website: www.annbrackenauthor.com

www.ingramcontent.com/pod-product-compliance
Lightning Source LLC
Chambersburg PA
CBHW031242290426
44109CB00012B/404